Food Safety

Other books in the At Issue series:

Affirmative Action
Are Efforts to Reduce Terrorism Successful?
Are the World's Coral Reefs Threatened?
Club Drugs
Do Animals Have Rights?
Does the World Hate the United States?
Do Infectious Diseases Pose a Serious Threat?
Do Nuclear Weapons Pose a Serious Threat?
The Ethics of Capital Punishment
The Ethics of Euthanasia
The Ethics of Genetic Engineering
The Ethics of Human Cloning
Fast Food
Gay and Lesbian Families
Gay Marriage
Gene Therapy
How Can School Violence Be Prevented?
How Should America's Wilderness Be Managed?
How Should the United States Withdraw from Iraq?
Internet Piracy
Is Air Pollution a Serious Threat to Health?
Is America Helping Afghanistan?
Is Gun Ownership a Right?
Is North Korea a Global Threat?
Is Racism a Serious Problem?
The Israeli-Palestinian Conflict
Media Bias
The Peace Movement
Reproductive Technology
Sex Education
Should Juveniles Be Tried as Adults?
Teen Suicide
Treating the Mentally Ill
UFOs
What Energy Sources Should Be Pursued?
What Motivates Suicide Bombers?
Women in the Military

Food Safety

Stuart A. Kallen, *Book Editor*

Bruce Glassman, *Vice President*
Bonnie Szumski, *Publisher*
Helen Cothran, *Managing Editor*

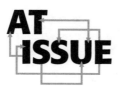 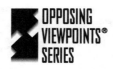

GREENHAVEN PRESS

An imprint of Thomson Gale, a part of The Thomson Corporation

THOMSON
GALE

Detroit • New York • San Francisco • San Diego • New Haven, Conn.
Waterville, Maine • London • Munich

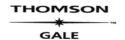

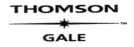

© 2005 Thomson Gale, a part of The Thomson Corporation.

Thomson and Star Logo are trademarks and Gale and Greenhaven Press are registered trademarks used herein under license.

For more information, contact
Greenhaven Press
27500 Drake Rd.
Farmington Hills, MI 48331-3535
Or you can visit our Internet site at http://www.gale.com

LIBRARY OF CONGRESS CATALOGING-IN-PUBLICATION DATA
Food safety / Stuart A. Kallen, book editor.
p. cm. — (At issue)
Includes bibliographical references and index.
ISBN 0-7377-2372-6 (lib. : alk. paper) — ISBN 0-7377-2373-4 (pbk. : alk. paper)
1. Food adulteration and inspection. 2. Food contamination. I. Kallen,
Stuart A., 1955– . II. At issue (San Diego, Calif.)
TX531.F5677 2005
363.19'2—dc22   2004052361

Printed in the United States of America

Contents

Page

Introduction 7

1. America's Food Supply Is Vulnerable to Agricultural 14
   Terrorism
   Jeff Greco

2. Federal Agencies Are Protecting America's Food 24
   Supply from Terrorists
   U.S. Food and Drug Administration

3. Genetically Engineered Crops Are Safe and Beneficial 33
   Gregory Conko and C.S. Prakash

4. Genetically Modified Food Has Great Potential 41
   for Harm
   Karen Charman

5. An Epidemic of Mad Cow Disease in the United 52
   States Is Inevitable
   Christine Wenc

6. Mad Cow Disease Is Not a Threat to the United States 63
   Elizabeth Whelan

7. Organic Food Is Expensive, Bad for the Environment, 67
   and Potentially Deadly
   Alex Knapp

8. More Americans Are Choosing Organic Food for 71
   Safety and Health
   Richard McGill Murphy

9. Irradiated Food Can Cause Cancer and Other 79
   Health Problems
   Public Citizen

10. Irradiation Makes the Food Supply Safer 87
    Robin Brett Parnes et al.

11. Pesticides in Foods Are Poisoning Consumers 96
    Charles M. Benbrook

12. Pesticides Are Rarely Dangerous and Provide   106
    Many Benefits
      Scott Phillips et al.

Organizations to Contact   114

Bibliography   118

Index   122

Introduction

With an astonishing 61 percent of adults in the United States considered overweight or obese, there is little doubt that Americans love to eat. Every year, the average American adult consumes more than 70 pounds of beef, 60 pounds of pork, 550 pounds of dairy products, 130 pounds of fruit, 142 pounds of potatoes, and 134 pounds of other vegetables. The average adult also ingests an incredible 152 pounds of refined sugar along with large quantities of flour, oil, and soda. Along with these foodstuffs, people take in about 10 pounds of chemical additives, including preservatives, flavoring and coloring agents, stabilizers, and drug and pesticide residues.

This vast quantity of food is supplied by a massive agribusiness industry consisting of farmers and ranchers, pesticide manufacturers, slaughterhouses, food producers, scientists, and researchers. The industry uses highly mechanized methods to raise, slaughter, and process tens of millions of cows, pigs, chickens, and other animals every year. The most modern scientific methods are used to harvest many of the grains, vegetables, and fruits that grace Americans' tables every day.

This cornucopia of food passes through more than fifty thousand food manufacturers, agricultural processors, and warehouses. To ensure the safety of this massive amount of food, inspectors for the U.S. Department of Agriculture (USDA) are appointed to inspect meat, poultry, and processed egg products, while the Food and Drug Administration (FDA) inspects all other foods.

While many take this amazing harvest for granted, a growing number of people are questioning just what it is that they are putting in their bodies, how it was raised, and how it ended up on their grocers' shelves. Consumers want to know if the foods they are eating are safe, and some feel that they have good reasons to wonder. According to a 1999 study conducted by *Consumer Reports* magazine, high levels of toxic pesticides such as methyl parathion and DDT—which is banned in the United States—were found on apples, grapes, green beans, peaches, pears, spinach, and winter squash. The study noted that "even a single daily serving of [this] produce can deliver unsafe levels of toxic pesticide residues for young children." Children exposed to these substances are at risk of suffering weakened immune systems, disrupted hormonal balances, and even brain damage.

Although the use of pesticides frightens some consumers, others argue that such fears are groundless. They point out that the safety level set for pesticides by the FDA is one hundred times lower than the level that might trigger cancer in a laboratory rat. According to agricultural analyst Dennis Avery, pesticides even play an important role in making Americans healthier:

> The FDA is convinced that pesticides help make fruits and vegetables more attractive, more widely available—and substantially cheaper. This greatly encourages fruit and vegetable consumption, especially in large families and poor families. That's vital, because the one-fourth of our population that eats the most produce has half the . . . cancer risk of the one-fourth that eats the least. No matter how the produce was grown. Fruit and vegetable consumption also lowers our risks of heart disease and brain dysfunction. For obvious reasons, the FDA thinks that protecting our fruits and vegetables with pesticides is important to the nation's health.

Because the FDA wants more vegetables available at the cheapest price, the agency also quickly approved the use of biotechnology; that is, genetically engineered (GE) fruits, vegetables, and grains. As with pesticides, however, the debate over the biotech food issue is heated.

The first GE food appeared in the United States in 1993 when scientists found a way to modify the genes in a tomato plant. In order to make the fruit ripen slower—and last longer on the way to market—scientists modified the plant's DNA. At the time, farmers were picking tomatoes when they were green and artificially ripening them off the vine by exposing them to ethylene gas in order to turn them red. These tomatoes were hard and tasteless. By contrast, GE "Flavr Savr" tomatoes were vine ripened and were said to be as tasty as those grown in consumers' own backyards. The main concern of the FDA was that the tomatoes might not be as nutritious as those grown using traditional methods. After industry tests confirmed that the Flavr Savr was equal to other tomatoes and that there were no increases in natural toxins due to the gene splicing, the FDA approved the tomato for sale. Soon tens of millions of consumers were buying and eating this genetically modified fruit without any knowledge that it was not a traditionally grown food.

In the years that followed, biotech researchers produced dozens of other GE foods. Some of these, such as corn and soybeans, have been modified so they can withstand massive amounts of pesticides that will kill weeds in the field without withering the crops. By 2001 more than half of the soybean crops and a quarter of the corn planted in the United States were genetically engineered. Since most corn and soybean crops are fed to animals, the meat and poultry that people eat is often derived from animals raised on genetically modified feed.

As the FDA never required GE foods to be labeled, few consumers thought about the safety of the new foods they were eating, which looked and tasted the same as traditional groceries. And these new products have proved to be extremely profitable for large agribusiness conglomerates such as Calgene and Monsanto.

By the late 1990s, however, there was a growing concern among researchers, advocates, and some consumers about the safety of GE foods. New scientific discoveries went far beyond ways to prevent tomatoes from ripening too quickly. Researchers started growing foods previously unimaginable. Some have produced corn that has pharmaceutical drugs such as animal vaccines implanted in the gene structure. Others have implanted insect, fish, pig, and human genes into fruits and vegetables. In most cases the stated reasons are to enhance herbicide resistance, reduce susceptibility to cold or frost, or increase the rates of growth. These new products have prompted consumer and environmental groups to call these transgenic crops "Frankenfoods," after the fictional monster—created by Dr. Frankenstein—that was built from body parts taken from several people. Reporter Peter Pringle listed the concerns of those opposed to GE or GM (genetically modified) foods in *Food, Inc.*:

> "Frankenfoods" . . . could cause allergies in humans and mutations in pests [that eat them]. They could produce agricultural monstrosities, such as invasive "superweeds" [immune to pesticides]. They could change the ecology of the planet in unpre-

dictable and irreversible ways. They could destroy biodiversity. They could even cause the extinction of important wild plants essential for breeding staple crops. GM [genetically modified] crops could destroy America's favorite insect, the monarch butterfly.

As these and other concerns over GE foods come to the attention of Americans, consumers have begun to voice doubts. A 2001 poll by the Center for Science in the Public Interest showed that 48 percent of shoppers would refuse to buy food if the label said it contained genetically altered ingredients. With this knowledge, the biotech industry continues to fight mandatory labeling of GE foods.

While genetic engineering and other concerns draw the attention of consumers and safe food advocates, Americans are often uninformed about other threats to their food supply—problems with far more immediate and dangerous consequences. According to the Centers for Disease Control (CDC), more than five thousand Americans die every year from food poisoning. In addition, a whopping 76 million are sickened and more than 325,000 become so ill that they must be hospitalized. Most of these cases are caused by a handful of foodborne pathogens including *Salmonella* and *E. coli*, which can sicken and kill those who ingest them. Those most affected are the elderly, young children, and pregnant women and their fetuses.

Critics argue that the agribusiness industry is not doing enough to prevent food poisoning. They point out that since the 1970s the food industry has grown into a centralized system of "factory farms," slaughterhouses, and agricultural processors where pathogens originating in the infected manure of one cow can spread from carcass to carcass until thousands of pounds of meat are contaminated. According to Caroline Smith DeWaal, the director of food safety at the Center for Science in the Public Interest, "Consumers play a lottery every day when they eat."

Although it is left to the USDA and FDA to prevent such outbreaks, critics point to many flaws in this system. In their report "Outbreak Alert," DeWaal and food safety researcher Kristina Barlow write:

> Although FDA-regulated foods are linked to two-thirds of outbreaks, the FDA's budget is just 31 percent of the total U.S. budget for food-safety in-

spections. Because of limited funding, the FDA inspects only 2 percent of the estimated 5 million shipments of imported food each year. And while meat-processing plants are inspected by USDA daily, plants processing seafood, eggs, produce, or processed foods containing less than 2 percent meat are inspected by FDA on average just once every five years. When foodborne-illness outbreaks do occur, neither the USDA nor the FDA has the power to order recalls of contaminated food. They must ask food companies to voluntarily remove foods from the market, which can delay the recall and increase the number of illnesses linked to an outbreak.

This low level of government involvement in the food supply has led to a new hazard in the last decade. According to industry critics, the unsanitary conditions found in huge slaughterhouses have created an environment that can also contribute to the spread of bovine spongiform encephalopathy, popularly known as BSE or mad cow disease. For reasons that remain unclear, this fearsome fatal disease that eats away the human brain developed when cows, which are herbivores, were given feed produced from rendered slaughterhouse waste products. Veterinarian and journalist Mark Jerome Walters describes this process in *Six Modern Plagues*:

> The term "rendering" is a euphemism for refining and repackaging animals' blood and guts into palatable feed for livestock. . . . [Meat] producers realized they could save money if they recycled and sold normally discarded by-products of butchered livestock, including the intestines, bladder, udder, kidneys, spleen, stomach, heart, liver, lungs, and other organs, as well as bones. Through the process of rendering, these leftovers could be turned back into feed for cattle, sheep, and other herbivores. Nature's plant-eaters could be transformed into human-made carnivores [and meat-eating cannibals].

This practice of giving cows rendered feed first came into question in Great Britain in 1986 when dozens of cows began drooling, staggering, and acting bizarrely aggressive. When these "mad cows" died, autopsies showed that their brains were spongy and filled with holes. Within a year at least 180,000 cows were diagnosed with mad cow disease, but an untold number of infected cows had already been butchered and eaten by consumers. Even as British farmers began the gruesome process of burning the carcasses of tens of thousands of diseased cattle, it was discovered that BSE can spread to people who eat the beef of infected cows. In humans, the disease mimics symptoms of a rare disorder called Creutzfeldt-Jakob disease (CJD), which researchers say infects about one in a million people. When BSE spread to people in England, the human version was called variant Creutzfeldt-Jakob disease, or vCJD. Unlike CJD, which only strikes the very old, vCJD attacks people of all ages.

One hundred thirty people have died from vCJD traced to mad cow disease, and the disorder continues to frighten knowledgeable scientists and consumers. It can take up to ten years before vCJD appears in infected people, and cows sick with BSE may not be detected among the millions of cattle slaughtered every week. This means that if BSE-infected meat has been sold to consumers, the USDA will not know about it for a decade.

Like other food safety issues, the mad cow scare has political implications. Consumer groups representing organic farmers, vegetarians, and environmentalists believe that BSE-tainted meat continues to make its way into the American food supply despite the ban on fattening cattle on rendered feed. These fears appeared justified in December 2003 when a single cow infected with BSE was found in Yakima, Washington. Groups such as the National Cattlemen's Beef Association defended their industry. They insisted that with USDA inspections, the American beef supply is one of the safest in the world. They also accused consumer advocates of exploiting what the cattlemen considered to be an isolated incident in order to attract attention to their own political agendas. As beef industry advocate Alex Avery writes:

> The coordinated lobbying efforts behind these food scares [is an] attempt to drive the American consumer into buying premium-priced "organic" and "natural" products. . . . But these campaigns aren't about facts and safety, they are about sales. For example, organic beef is not any safer from Mad Cow disease than non-organic beef, despite the higher price, because the entire U.S. food system is equally well protected.

With millions of pounds of beef being processed in a handful of huge slaughterhouses every day, many critics feel concerned about the safety of this popular food. They point out that twice as many people die every year from food poisoning as were killed in the September 11, 2001, terrorist attack on the World Trade Center.

Despite fears about food safety, eating remains one of humanity's oldest pleasures. In the United States, with the most abundant and varied food supply in the world, most people give little thought to the farming and processing methods behind their daily bread. But when disaster strikes—from whatever source—they expect the government, scientists, and industry to protect their food supply. In a modern industrialized world with an ever-growing population, however, there will always be new risks, new threats, and new solutions devised in order to feed the masses. This reality is reflected in the arguments put forth in the following pages. In *At Issue: Food Safety* the authors present differing views on the food people eat, how it is grown and processed, and how safe and healthful it is for consumers.

1

America's Food Supply Is Vulnerable to Agricultural Terrorism

Jeff Greco

Jeff Greco is a policy analyst with the Midwestern Office of the Council of State Governments and a staff member of the Midwestern Legislative Conference's Agricultural Committee.

American agriculture is extremely vulnerable to terrorist attack. The U.S. government has only just begun to address the threat to farms and food processing plants and still has few plans in place to deal with an agricultural catastrophe. If terrorists are able to contaminate food supplies at large, centralized meat processing plants, tens of thousands of people could sicken or die. Such an attack would seriously threaten the multi-billion dollar food industry and could result in severe food shortages. An agroterrorist attack could disrupt the country's livestock and grain supply and have grave consequences that would rival those of the September 11, 2001, attacks on the World Trade Center and the Pentagon.

Terrorism is not an easy concept to define. After Sept. 11 [2001], many Americans were forced to broaden their understanding of terrorism to include non-state-sponsored acts motivated by religious or issue-based extremism rather than ideology. The subsequent anthrax attacks, by employing a biological agent to provoke a public response more typical of a physical attack, further shaped public perceptions of terrorism.

Jeff Greco, "Agricultural Terrorism in the Midwest: Risks, Threats, and State Responses," Council of State Governments, Midwestern Office, www.csgmidwest. org, December 2002. Copyright © 2002 by the Council of State Governments. Reproduced with permission.

One reason why agricultural terrorism may ultimately prove attractive to terrorists is the novelty of the approach.

Most forms of agroterror lurk at the fringe of what society has typically defined as terrorism and may again catch many Americans by surprise if and when an attack occurs. The classical definition of terrorism—the use of violence and intimidation to achieve an end—may not entirely apply when agricultural targets are selected, especially if no human lives are lost as a consequence. But terrorism also involves an element of fear and quantifiable losses, both of which would soon emerge in the aftermath of a large-scale attack.

Studies in Conflict and Terrorism, a periodical whose editors and contributors have discussed the agroterror phenomenon for many years, defines agricultural terrorism as the "infiltration and destruction of a society's food source through the contamination of livestock or the sabotage of grains." This formulation captures both the psychological impact of an attack—the loss of food sources that are critical to human sustenance—as well as the devastating economic impact of such an attack.

Understanding the threat

While investigators, health authorities and the public struggle to understand and respond appropriately to an agroterror event, the event itself can quickly spiral out of control. One classic case worth noting is the suspected poisoning of Chilean grapes in 1989; despite repeated threats of cyanide contamination, no poisoning was ever found, no one became ill, and no evidence of an actual attack ever surfaced. Yet panicked consumers refused to buy Chilean fruit of any kind—and suppliers declined to stock it—and the Chilean agriculture industry lost an estimated $210 million from the incident.

During the [2001] foot-and-mouth-disease outbreak in the United Kingdom, the British agriculture industry's staggering losses were compounded by a decline in tourism, the skepticism of foreign markets toward British farm products of any kind, and the loss of confidence on the part of agricultural producers toward the British government that cannot be quantified. While not an act of terror, the crisis nevertheless illustrated how unconventional acts of terror could have vast and unpredictable consequences.

No one died as a result of the 2001 outbreak of foot-and-mouth disease, but it did result in billions of dollars in damage.

Likewise, most acts of agroterrorism are unlikely to involve large numbers of human fatalities, but the effects could still be devastating.

One way to reduce the agroterror threat is simply to raise awareness of the nature of the threat—and to do so in a way that does not dismiss the reality that the long-term consequences of such an event are every bit as serious (if not more so) as those of a more conventional terrorist attack.

> *Some biological agents are easy to manipulate and may appeal more to amateur terrorists with little experience in planning complicated attacks.*

A broader public conception of terrorism that includes "nonviolent" agroterror events could better prepare the public for an attack, which, in turn, could mitigate the consequences by ensuring a more effective response. The conventional definition of terrorism as the use of violence to achieve a political goal is simply too narrow to encompass the specter of agricultural terror, which relies on psychological intimidation (and often violence toward animals) to achieve its objectives.

Why agriculture is at risk

Clearly, there are higher-profile, more attractive targets available to terrorists than agricultural property and holdings.

As noted above, some perpetrators may also be disappointed to discover that biological weapons in general, and agricultural terrorism in particular, are not an efficient way of producing large-scale human casualties. But a human tragedy is not always the only outcome terrorists are willing to accept; indeed, some terrorists may fear that a surplus of human fatalities would harm them or their cause.

Rand Corporation terrorism expert Peter Chalk notes that environmental activists, who have been responsible for the majority of recent agroterror incidents (as well as threats), are also keen to build public support for their cause, raise funds and cultivate a positive image among certain segments of the public—tasks that are undermined by human injuries or fatalities.

Chalk cites fellow Rand terrorism expert Bruce Hoffman:

"Agricultural terrorism (conveys) a coercive point but doesn't necessarily cross the threshold of killing people, and thus doesn't create the same kind of backlash."

Opponents of genetically modified crops, animal exploitation, or U.S. food and land policies have already caused substantial damage to facilities in several Midwestern and Pacific Northwest states, and as these movements gain strength, terrorism analysts expect a comparable increase in such incidents.

In addition, certain perpetrators may be more reticent to jeopardize their own lives and health for the sake of their cause, and agricultural targets involve much less risk to the perpetrators themselves. Finally, some biological agents are easy to manipulate and may appeal more to amateur terrorists with little experience in planning complicated attacks.

Agroterror is a threat to jobs, food supply

The USDA's [United States Department of Agriculture's] 1997 Census of Agriculture estimates that the nation's agriculture industry pumps $1.3 trillion into the economy, more than $200 billion of which is in the form of raw agricultural produce. . . . While no attack could destroy the entire agricultural industry—which constitutes 13 percent of the gross domestic product—even a small-scale incident could result in massive losses.

The recent foot-and-mouth epidemic in the UK is again instructive: although the outbreak was short and the response efficient, the USDA reports that the British government was still forced to slaughter some 11 million animals at a cost of more than $10 billion to the British economy in compensation paid to farmers. (The indirect costs to the tourism and retail industries are even greater.)

According to Chalk, the indirect costs of an attack, though often incalculable, are usually far higher. When avian influenza hit portions of the U.S. poultry industry in 1983–1984, for example, the eradication cost of $63 million was dwarfed by the estimated $349 million rise in poultry product prices to consumers in the first six months of the outbreak. . . .

The simultaneous contamination of several livestock facilities could shut down the nation's food distribution system, force the destruction of a large portion of the country's livestock industry (through mass cullings), and result in the layoffs of thousands of feedlot workers and food processors. Any positive disease reading would likely trigger an international embargo of U.S. food products, about 24 percent of which are exported annually. In the Midwest, some $20 billion in farm exports are at risk.

An especially large-scale attack also could threaten food supplies; an April 2001 study by the College of Staten Island, New York, claims that "the average U.S. city has a five-day supply of fresh meat, fruit, and vegetables . . . a risk made more acute as many urban supermarkets no longer rely on large in-store inventories, but instead depend on just-in-time deliveries." In the Midwest—where agriculture employs up to 25 percent of the workforce in states such as Kansas, Nebraska and the Dakotas, and where cash receipts for farm products amount to $4 billion to $9 billion annually per state—even a minor disruption in agricultural commerce could cost thousands of jobs and millions of dollars in lost income.

The ongoing consolidation of U.S. agricultural facilities and assets is of particular concern. Larger facilities not only render an attack easier to execute, they also exacerbate the impact of a terrorist event if animals in close proximity to each other spread a biological or chemical agent easily.

Michael Dunn, a bioterrorism expert at the New York Academy of Sciences, estimates that by 2010, just 30 feedlots will generate 50 percent of the country's slaughtered cattle, a typical poultry farm will have more than 1 million birds, and feedlots of 500,000 cattle will not be uncommon. While consolidated facilities give producers and regulators an opportunity to tighten security in ways that might not be practical at large numbers of smaller facilities, the potential impact of a security breach is nevertheless alarming.

> *Larger facilities not only render an attack easier to execute, they also exacerbate the impact of a terrorist event.*

Dunn suggests that the transfer of animals between feedlots, along with the mixing of animals from different feedlots at slaughterhouses, is becoming more common. This increases the likelihood that even a small-scale attack would have at least regional, rather than merely local, implications, he believes.

The regional impact of an attack could be especially devastating given the lack of diversity in much of the U.S. agricultural industry.

Most states' farm economies depend on just a few—even one or two—agricultural products; likewise, the country often receives its entire supply of a particular food from one region or state. The concentration of cattle in western Kansas and neighboring areas, for example, not only makes it much easier for a terrorist to wipe out an entire region's economy, but also makes it easier to effectively wipe out a large portion of an entire industry on which the nation depends. A carefully targeted attack on several commodities could decimate large swaths of the U.S. farm economy and severely diminish the nation's food supply.

Finally, terrorists might well target agriculture simply because of its vulnerability. At a time when the security of other potential targets has been increased, agriculture may be one of the few areas of vulnerability left exposed. Armed with a minimum of scientific knowledge and equipment, a terrorist can introduce devastating diseases with little or no risk of getting caught—or getting the disease.

"The critical issue with agroterrorism," according to a 2001 Purdue University report on the issue, "is the low level of technical knowledge required to use it in some cases. Any person with minimal understanding of microbiology can acquire the organisms and spread them."

Why hasn't an agroterror attack happened yet?

The relative ease with which an agroterror attack can be launched raises the question of why such events are so rare. Some policymakers argue that the lack of a high-profile, successful agroterror event suggests that large-scale attacks are difficult to perpetrate, and therefore less deserving of government attention and resources. But, in fact, agroterrorism is nothing new, and technological advances have actually made carrying out such attacks easier in recent years.

According to the FBI, more than 500 acts of environmental terrorism have occurred in the United States over the past five years, although some of these incidents did not involve direct contamination of the food supply. Many of these acts escaped public attention either because they did not fall within common understandings of what terrorism is or because authorities prevented the attack from seriously endangering the public. But each of these incidents—ranging from a May 2001 contamination of an Oregon tree farm by environmental extremists to the destruction of genetically modified corn in California in 1999—represents an assault on the integrity of the U.S. agriculture industry. No matter how trivial, each incident reinforces an impression of vulnerability that might eventually elicit larger-scale attacks by groups with a greater capacity to inflict real damage to the industry.

> *With more than 500,000 farms and 57,000 processors in the United States, and more than 350,000 acres of farmland in the Midwest alone, no inspection regime could fully guarantee safety and security.*

While many of the more recent attacks targeted agribusiness personnel and infrastructure rather than the general food supply, there is plenty of evidence that the food supply is vulnerable. In a well-known 1984 incident, more than 700 individuals in northern Oregon fell ill when members of the Rajneesh cult contaminated restaurant salad bars with salmonella; similar incidents, with fewer victims, have occurred several times since then. In 2000, 27 people in Quebec were poisoned with arsenic from a single coffee machine. During both world wars, combatant states targeted livestock and/or crops—anthrax was among the agents used—with little overall effect.

Within the last several years, activists have destroyed experimental crops in such diverse locales as Italy, New Zealand and several U.S. states. Recent incidents have included attacks on crops grown by the University of California, the University of Washington and, in the Midwest, Michigan State University. While no proof was ever discovered, groups have also claimed responsibility for natural disasters as well: a 1989 fly infestation in southern California and a 1996 outbreak of citrus canker in Florida (the latter was attributed to the Cuban biological weapons program).

Yet, in the past, few policymakers have considered such incidents a threat to national security; local media reports in the Oregon and Quebec cases did not even describe the attacks as a form of terrorism. When attacks are seen as the work of isolated groups or unstable individuals, implications may seem inconsequential. But in the post–Sept. 11 [2001] world, no attack—no matter how minor—will escape extensive media scrutiny. . . .

The food production process is vulnerable

The key vulnerability of the U.S. agriculture industry is the diffuse nature of its holdings. Unlike other potential targets—the nuclear power industry, border zones, military sites, etc., which have relatively concentrated holdings that can be more easily guarded and defended—millions of acres of agricultural land and thousands of processing facilities are too numerous to fully monitor.

Contamination of foodstuffs can occur at any point during the food production process, from the importation of seeds to the unpacking of finished products at a supermarket. Along the way, even relatively unprocessed food passes through warehouses and packaging/labeling facilities and is transported several times on vehicles that are not always secure. Harvard University microbiology researcher Rocco Casagrande notes that vastly different kinds of attacks—on various commodities, using various agents and in various kinds of facilities—gives the potential terrorist many options from which to choose.

"The two extremes" of "crops that are grown over thousands of square miles" and "a modern animal farm with often several hundred thousand animals in one location . . . require that a terrorist use markedly different techniques." Diverse vulnerabilities also pose a challenge to law enforcement, emergency management personnel, government regulators and producers aiming to prevent and/or respond to agroterror attacks.

> *The plausibility and appeal of such an attack are now beyond question.*

In light of such difficulties, complete surveillance of U.S. agriculture holdings is not a realistic, cost-effective objective. With more than 500,000 farms and 57,000 processors in the United States, and more than 350,000 acres of farmland in the Midwest alone, no inspection regime could fully guarantee safety and security.

Risk management is critical. By focusing on key vulnerabilities, industry and government leaders can significantly reduce the likelihood of an attack as well as the severity of damage if an attack does occur; smaller sites with fewer animals may be harder to secure, but the consequences of an attack may also be constrained.

As the agricultural industry consolidates, and as fewer and fewer farmers and facilities control an ever-larger percentage of the nation's agricultural output, the range of attractive targets narrows. This consolidation is a double-edged sword in the fight against agroterror: it limits the scope of damage at minor facilities and small farms, but it dramatically expands the range and reach of terrorists who are able to penetrate larger packing plants and processing facilities. [Terrorism expert] Chalk contends that "the outbreak of a contagious disease (at a large facility) would be very difficult to control and could necessitate the destruction of all the livestock, a formidable and expensive task.". . .

Different kinds of attacks

Direct attacks on crops or livestock would be economically devastating to producers and the industry, especially if mass cullings, vaccinations or economic sanctions followed. But the impact on public health might be limited—as, for example, the British outbreak of foot-and-mouth disease was in 2001—if state authorities could identify the problem before contaminated food products reached consumers. On the other hand, an attack during a later stage of the food production process might occur too late to prevent human illness and/or death. This kind of attack might have more limited consequences for the industry if the origin of the contamination could be quickly identified, since the chief assets of the agriculture industry (crops, livestock, most facilities) would be undamaged. But a large-scale human tragedy would shake public confidence in the safety and security of U.S. agriculture, disrupt the nation's efficient food supply system and depress sales of U.S. produce for the foreseeable future.

In both cases, the economic damage is significant, but the public health component of a later-stage attack adds a critical, emotional element that may make recovery more difficult. This report, however, focuses primarily on pre-harvest risks to producers and their assets, since this segment of the agriculture industry may be less attuned to security issues than later-stage processors that have faced security crises on a more regular basis. Nevertheless, it bears repeating that a security breach at any stage of the food production process would have severe repercussions for the industry as a whole; security is a collective responsibility that producers, processors, retailers and regulators should mutually enforce. . . .

Systematic efforts to combat the threat of agricultural terrorism are still in their infancy. The attacks of Sept. 11, 2001, along with the 2001 foot-and-mouth-disease crisis in the UK, did focus the attention of the U.S. agricultural community on the threat, and most states have begun to address it in concrete ways. The plausibility and appeal of such an attack are now beyond question, and industry leaders have worked hard to demonstrate the potentially devastating impact of even a relatively minor agroterror event in the current climate of global uncertainty.

But poor communication between government agencies, between levels of government, and between the public and private sectors continue to hinder states in their efforts to adopt a seamless approach to agricultural terrorism preparedness and prevention.

Many states do not yet recognize agricultural terrorism as a legally distinct phenomenon, complicating the prosecution of perpetrators, the swift response of emergency action teams, and surveillance and inspection efforts. In other cases, the facilities and procedures that animal health, emergency management and other agencies have at their disposal are not yet equipped to deal with the intentional spread of dangerous diseases. Laboratories are unable to test for exotic diseases and too few in number to cope with a major crisis, while personnel are not trained to identify security risks or to diagnose foreign animal diseases.

Antiquated reporting systems in many areas delay transmission of vital disease vectors among veterinarians and producers; and regulations that require producers and veterinarians to share security information, emergency plans and positive disease diagnoses with state authorities are either not enforced or do not exist at all. Many important changes will require an institutional shift in thinking among producers, responders and legislators that the events of Sept. 11 [2001] have already set in motion. The challenge for industry leaders and regulators is to take the necessary steps to secure the U.S. agricultural sector before another such tragedy occurs.

2

Federal Agencies Are Protecting America's Food Supply from Terrorists

U.S. Food and Drug Administration

The U.S. Food and Drug Administration oversees the safety and regulation of about 80 percent of the American food supply.

Since the terrorist attacks of September 11, 2001, the U.S. Food and Drug Administration (FDA) has spent millions of dollars to protect the nation's food supply. The FDA has developed programs to prevent an attack on the food supply, respond in the event that an attack does take place, and recover quickly from any threats. While agroterrorism remains a menace, the government is hard at work to protect and monitor farms, feedlots, and food processors.

The [terrorist] events of September 11, 2001, heightened the nation's awareness and placed a renewed focus on ensuring the protection of the nation's critical infrastructures. A terrorist attack on the food supply could pose both severe public health and economic impacts, while damaging the public's confidence in the food we eat. Several food incidents since the fall of 2001 highlight the significance of FDA's [Food and Drug Administration] food security activities. In the fall of 2002, a competitor of a restauranteur in China added a chemical com-

U.S. Food and Drug Administration, "Progress Report to Secretary Tommy G. Thompson: Ensuring the Safety and Security of the Nation's Food Supply," www.cfsan.fda.gov, July 23, 2003.

pound to his competitor's food and killed dozens of people and sent hundreds more to hospitals. Also in the fall of 2002, three individuals were arrested in Jerusalem for allegedly planning to carry out a mass poisoning of patrons at a local café. One of the arrested individuals worked as a chef at the café. In January 2003, several individuals were arrested in Britain for plotting to add [the poison] ricin to the food supply on a British military base. Each of these incidents shows the potential for the nation's food supply to be used in an attack.

> *U.S. borders are flooded with FDA-regulated imports from all over the world.*

Even before September 11, HHS [Department of Health and Human Services] was taking steps to improve food security. As part of the initial response to these heightened concerns after September 11, Congress provided FDA with new statutory authorities and some additional resources for food inspection. As a result of new threats to the food supply and new opportunities, FDA has made fundamental changes in how we implement our mission of protecting our food supply, so that all Americans can have confidence that their foods are not only safe but also secure. . . .

FDA food security strategy

In the months before and after Sept. 11, 2001, [HHS] Secretary [Tommy G.] Thompson led the effort to encourage Congress to increase FDA funding to protect the nation's families from an attack on the food supply. In fiscal years 2002 and 2003, Congress enacted more than $195 million for food safety programs, allowing FDA to hire 655 new food personnel and conduct more than double the previous number of food import examinations. In President Bush's fiscal year 2004 budget, the Department of Health and Human Services is requesting $116.3 million, an increase of $20.5 million over 2003, to further protect the nation's food supply.

The agency is employing overall strategies to (1) develop increased awareness among federal, state, local, and tribal governments and the private sector by collecting, analyzing, and disseminating information and knowledge (Awareness); (2) develop capacity for identification of a specific threat or attack on the food supply (Prevention); (3) develop effective protection strategies to "shield" the food supply from terrorist threats (Preparedness); (4) develop capacity for rapid, coordinated response to a foodborne terrorist attack (Response); and (5) develop capacity for rapid, coordinated recovery from a foodborne terrorist attack (Recovery). . . .

FDA has worked and continues to work closely with the states and other food safety, law enforcement, and intelligence agencies to collaborate on research, emergency response, and information exchange, all of which significantly strengthen the nation's food safety and security system.

In the wake of September 11, 2001 . . . FDA moved expeditiously and quickly to establish this additional investigative and scientific team by rapidly hiring and training 655 additional field personnel. Of the 655, 97% are allocated to food safety field activities: 300 support the conduct of consumer safety investigations at U.S. ports of entry, 100 support laboratory analyses on imported products, 33 are for criminal investigations of import activities, and the remaining personnel support domestic efforts.

The Public Health Security and Bioterrorism Preparedness and Response Act (Bioterrorism Act) was enacted in June 2002 and by the end of the year, FDA had started to place additional, trained investigators and analysts at targeted locations. Training of these new personnel has been paramount. . . .

> *Since 2001, FDA more than quintupled the number of food import examinations.*

U.S. borders are flooded with FDA-regulated imports from all over the world, and the continuous threat of terrorism requires FDA to remain vigilant in its effort to retain a competent, trained workforce if we are to maintain a high level of readiness. With FDA's limited resources to meet the challenge of assuring the food safety and security for more than 6 million entries per year, FDA must strategically develop hiring, targeting resources and succession planning to be prepared in the event of a terrorist attack.

Mobilizing new staff

FDA not only mobilized new staff but redirected, trained current investigators and scientists to integrate and strengthen its food safety and security mission and ensured that the agency has the necessary scientific and logistical expertise to respond to an event that could threaten the safety and security of the food supply. FDA has hired or re-trained scientific experts in biological, chemical, and radiological agent research, detection methodology, preventive technologies and acquired substantial knowledge of these agents to help support domestic and import activities. FDA's Office of Regulatory Affairs (ORA) has developed a succession plan to ensure that the agency will continue to have highly trained and competent scientists, investigators, analysts, and managers to accomplish the agency's overall mission of consumer protection. FDA realizes that recruitment and retention of our highly skilled and sometimes very specialized workforce requires thoughtful planning so that we will be ready to effectively and efficiently meet the future challenges FDA faces.

Imports—a strategic approach

FDA continues to adjust its import program via the development of an Import Strategic Plan (ISP) to reflect the changing nature of risks and trade associated with imported goods. This approach encompasses and addresses the full "life-cycle" of imported products. As part of the ISP, FDA is assessing information derived from foreign and domestic inspectional operations, adverse events, consumer complaints, recall activities, and information technology. The goal of the ISP is to better protect the public health and safety by decreasing the risk that unsafe, ineffective, or violative products will enter U.S. commerce through our borders, ports, and other import hubs. Moreover, when implemented, the ISP will provide FDA with the critical flexibility it needs to shift resources as import trends alter the risks and change priorities for public health and safety protection.

Historically, the volume of U.S. imports of FDA-regulated products was relatively small and consisted of raw ingredients and bulk materials intended for further processing or incorporation into finished products. Therefore, FDA could rely more heavily on physical examination and domestic inspections to ensure that imported raw ingredients and bulk materials were properly handled, received, quarantined, released, and processed according to good manufacturing practices and sanitation principles.

Even with the recent increases of personnel for counterterrorism efforts, border inspections cannot manage the changes in the nature of risks and trade. FDA is taking steps to implement a risk-based approach towards covering the importation of FDA-regulated goods. These proactive steps will assist FDA in identifying patterns of transportation while goods are in international streams of commerce; increase our ability to conduct effective, efficient foreign inspections; and will aid FDA in making admissibility decisions before goods enter domestic commerce. Moreover, the risk-based approaches we are contemplating include exploring the feasibility of forming regulatory partnerships to provide better information to FDA—and, ultimately, better protection to U.S. consumers.

> *FDA increased joint activities with federal, state, and local partners to help ensure a safe and secure food supply.*

FDA is supporting this enhanced import strategic plan by providing a greater import presence at our nation's borders. FDA is enhancing our capacity and capability to perform normal import operations such as sample collection and analysis, field examinations, and inspections across all our programs. In 2001, FDA provided coverage at about 40 ports of entry. By 2002, FDA had more than doubled its presence to 90 ports of entry.

In addition, since 2001, FDA more than quintupled the number of food import examinations. In 2001, FDA conducted 12,000 food exams. FDA has conducted over 62,000 food exams already this fiscal year and has surpassed its 2003 year-end goal of 48,000 food exams. This increased coverage was due to redirecting resources dedicated to assure increased import coverage during Operation Liberty Shield when the nation was at a heightened security alert. . . .

Bioterrorism Act regulations

FDA is on schedule to publish four major new regulations in accordance with provisions of the Bioterrorism Act. . . . These

rules implement new authority that FDA received in the Bioterrorism Act and are one of the most significant enhancements
of FDA's statutory authority to keep food imports secure.

On February 3, 2003, FDA and the Department of Treasury
jointly published in the *Federal Register* a proposed regulation[1]
implementing the provisions in the Bioterrorism Act that
would require owners, operators, or agents of a foreign or domestic facility where food is manufactured/processed, packed,
or held to submit a registration to FDA that includes basic information about the facility, emergency contact information,
and the categories of food the facility handles.

On February 3, 2003, FDA and the Department of Treasury
also jointly published in the *Federal Register* a proposed regulation[2] implementing the provisions in the Bioterrorism Act that
would require FDA to receive prior notice before imported food
arrives at the U.S. port of arrival.

On May 9, 2003, FDA published in the *Federal Register* a proposed regulation[3] implementing the provisions in the Bioterrorism Act that would require manufacturers, processors, pack-
ers, transporters, distributors, receivers, holders, and importers
of food to keep records identifying the immediate previous
source from which they receive food, as well as the immediate
subsequent recipient, to whom they sent food. . . .

Operation Liberty Shield

In March 2003, the United States government launched Operation Liberty Shield to increase security and readiness in the
United States at a time of elevated risk for a terrorist attack. Operation Liberty Shield, a comprehensive national plan of action
to protect many of America's critical infrastructures, was a uni-
fied operation coordinated by the Department of Homeland
Security that integrated selected national protective measures
with the involvement and support of federal, state, local, and
private responders and authorities from around the country.
Operation Liberty Shield was designed to provide increased
protection for America's citizens and infrastructure while main-
taining the free flow of goods and people across our border
with minimal disruption to our economy and way of life. FDA
has established protocols, trained staff and deployed supplies

1. The regulation has now taken effect.   2. The regulation has now taken effect.
3. The regulation has not yet taken effect.

and equipment for future and similar elevated threat level actions. A key component of Operation Liberty Shield was increasing and targeting surveillance of both domestic and imported food. The agency initiated the following activities:

- FDA issued new industry guidance documents on security measures and encouraged industry to voluntarily assess their security measures in response to an increased threat level. . . .
- FDA held a series of conference calls to brief state regulatory agencies, industry trade associations, consumer groups, and their federal counterparts, on Operation Liberty Shield and to request their assistance in distributing the food security guidance documents to domestic facilities and the portion of the import community that handles food products.
- FDA increased its surveillance of the domestic food industry, during Operation Liberty Shield, by conducting 844 inspections of domestic firms based on risk/threat assessments with a focus on enhancing awareness of food security at these facilities by providing copies of appropriate food security guidance documents. These investigations targeted examinations of specific commodities based on risk/threat assessments and sampled specific commodities based on risk/threat.
- FDA increased its monitoring of imported foods, during Operation Liberty Shield, by conducting increased examinations of specific imported commodities based on FDA's risk/threat assessments; enhancing the import communities' awareness of food security at ports by providing copies of FDA's food security guidance documents and sampling imported foods based on risk/threat assessments. FDA collected and analyzed 387 import samples for chemical and microbiological contaminants.
- FDA conducted domestic and import reconciliation exams to confirm that regulated commodities were what they purported to be, exposed unexplained differences between associated documentation and the product, and uncovered signs of tampering or counterfeiting.
- FDA increased joint activities with federal, state, and local partners to help ensure a safe and secure food supply, including working with the Centers for Disease Control and Prevention to ensure that outbreaks or unusual patterns of illness or injury are quickly investigated.

- Likewise, USDA [U.S. Department of Agriculture] undertook similar food security measures and activities for its regulated industries including meat, poultry, and processed egg products. Thus, in combination, FDA and USDA comprehensively covered the U.S. food supply. . . .

Dedicated to ensuring safety

FDA through its aggressive program, has made significant progress in strengthening the safety and security of the nation's food supply.

Nearly 20% of all imports into the U.S. are food and food products. FDA anticipates that we will receive over 8 million food shipments from over 200,000 foreign manufacturers this year—a huge volume that continues to grow rapidly. To meet this challenge, FDA is providing a greater import presence. FDA has placed an additional 300 field personnel at U.S. ports of entry. FDA now has a presence at 90 ports of entry and quintupled the number of food import examinations it performed this year compared to 2001—FDA has exceeded its year-end goal of 48,000 by 14,000 food import examinations.

FDA is using risk-based strategies to provide better information and in its collaborative efforts with other entities. This includes working with foreign authorities and manufacturers to improve production and shipping practices abroad as an alternative to detailed inspections at the border. FDA is using better information on imports to focus border checks on products that present significant potential risks and is working with producers to improve checks on the integrity of ingredients and to implement common-sense steps to reduce security risks.

FDA is on schedule to publish four major new regulations in accordance with provisions of the Bioterrorism Act that provide the agency with most significant enhancements to FDA's statutory authority to keep food imports secure. The agency intends to publish two final rules in October [2003] and two additional final rules by the end of [2003].

FDA has taken unprecedented steps to develop food security research. FDA has received $5 million in supplemental funding from OMB [Office of Management and Budget] to support FDA's food security research iniative. FDA is using this supplemental funding to focus on three broad areas: development of prevention and mitigation technologies and strategies, elucidation of agent characteristics, and development of means for continuously assessing foods for contamination. FDA has redirected existing research staff to focus on key priority issues and has over 25 intramural research projects ongoing related to food security. FDA is developing a broader research agenda to address critical research needs to aggressively meet food security challenges.

FDA remains dedicated to ensuring the safety and security of the nation's food supply. Americans depend on FDA to keep food safe and secure, and FDA will keep doing all we can to fulfill this critical mission.

3

Genetically Engineered Crops Are Safe and Beneficial

Gregory Conko and C.S. Prakash

Gregory Conko and C.S. Prakash are the cofounders of the AgBioWorld Foundation, a nonprofit organization that provides information to the public about developments in plant science, biotechnology, and sustainable agriculture.

Food that has been genetically modified can end hunger, provide improved nutritional quality, and allow farmers to use fewer pesticides. These benefits are particularly important to people living in impoverished developing nations. Those who claim that agricultural biotechnology is unsafe for human health and the environment ignore the merits of genetically engineered (GE) food. While Americans have the luxury of criticizing GE food, many people in India, China, and elsewhere need it to survive.

D uring the coming decades the world will face the extraordinary challenge of conquering poverty and achieving genuine food security with a very potent new tool: agricultural biotechnology. Skeptics argue that transgenic plants represent a vast new threat to both the environment and human health. However, that view is not supported by the overwhelming weight of scientific evidence that has been generated over the last three decades. Furthermore, such criticism ignores the fact that needless restrictions on biotechnology could endanger our ability to battle hunger in the 21st century.

Gregory Conko and C.S. Prakash, "Battling Hunger with Biotechnology," *Economic Perspectives*, vol. 7, May 1, 2002. Mr. Conko is a Senior Fellow at the Competitive Enterprise Institute. Dr. Prakash is a Professor of Plant Molecular Genetics at Tuskegee University. Reproduced with permission of the authors.

Transgenic technology holds the potential to increase food production, reduce the use of synthetic chemical pesticides, and actually make foods safer and healthier. These advances are critical in a world where natural resources are finite and where one-and-a-half billion people suffer from hunger and malnutrition. Already, farmers in the United States, Canada, and elsewhere have benefited from improvements in productivity and reduced use of synthetic pesticides. But the real future of biotechnology lies in addressing the special problems faced by farmers in less developed nations.

Critics like to dismiss such claims as nothing more than corporate public relations puffery. However, while most commercially available biotech plants were designed for farmers in the industrialized world, the increasing adoption of transgenic varieties by developing countries over the past few years has been remarkable. According to the International Service for the Acquisition of Agri-Biotech Applications (ISAAA), farmers in less developed countries now grow nearly one-quarter of the world's transgenic crops on more than 26 million acres (10.7 million hectares), and they do so for many of the same reasons that farmers in industrialized nations do.

> *In China . . . some 400 to 500 cotton farmers die every year from acute pesticide poisoning.*

Among the most important limiting factors in developing world agricultural productivity is biotic stress from insects, weeds, and plant diseases. Transgenic modifications common in several industrialized nations target these same problems and can be easily transferred into local varieties to help poor farmers in the developing world. For example, South African farmers are already growing transgenic pest-resistant maize, and this year [2002], began planting transgenic soy. South African and Chinese farmers have been growing transgenic insect-resistant cotton for several years, and the Indian government approved it for commercial cultivation in the spring of 2002. This transgenic cotton, similar to the varieties so popular in the United States, is expected to boost yields by 30 percent or more for Indian farmers, according to a recent article in the *Economic Times*. It could even transform India from the world's third largest producer of cotton into the largest.

Globally, transgenic varieties are now grown on more than 109 million acres (44.2 million hectares) in Argentina, Australia, Canada, Chile, China, Mexico, South Africa, and the United States, according to ISAAA. They are even grown on substantial amounts of acreage in Brazil, where no transgenic varieties have yet been approved for commercial cultivation. Farmers there looked across the border and saw how well their Argentine neighbors were doing with transgenic varieties, and smuggling of transgenic soybean seed became rampant. The European Union's (EU) Directorate General for Agriculture estimates that Brazil is now the fifth largest grower of transgenic crops.

Meeting environmental goals

Although this first generation of crops was designed primarily to improve farming efficiency, the environmental benefits these crops offer are extensive. The U.S. Department of Agriculture [USDA] found that U.S. farmers growing transgenic pest-resistant cotton, maize, and soy reduced the total volume of insecticides and herbicides they sprayed by more than 8 million pounds per year. Similar reductions have been seen in Canada with transgenic rapeseed [used for canola oil], according to the Canola Council of Canada.

In less developed nations where pesticides are typically sprayed on crops by hand, transgenic pest-resistant crops have had even greater benefits. In China, for example, some 400 to 500 cotton farmers die every year from acute pesticide poisoning. A study conducted by researchers at Rutgers University in the United States and the Chinese Academy of Sciences [in Taipei] found that adoption of transgenic cotton varieties in China has lowered the amount of pesticides used by more than 75 percent and reduced the number of pesticide poisonings by an equivalent amount. Another study by economists at the University of Reading in Britain found that South African cotton farmers have seen similar benefits.

The reduction in pesticide spraying also means that fewer natural resources are consumed to manufacture and transport the chemicals. Researchers at Auburn University and Louisiana State University in the United States found that, in 2000 alone, U.S. farmers growing transgenic cotton used 2.4 million fewer gallons of fuel, 93 million fewer gallons of water, and were spared some 41,000 10-hour days needed to apply pesticide sprays.

Transgenic herbicide-tolerant crops have promoted the adoption of farming practices that reduce tillage or eliminate it altogether. Low-tillage practices can decrease soil erosion by up to 90 percent compared to conventional cultivation, saving valuable topsoil, improving soil fertility, and dramatically reducing sedimentation in lakes, ponds, and waterways.

The productivity gains generated by transgenic crops provide yet another important environmental benefit: they could save millions of hectares of sensitive wildlife habitat from being converted into farmland. The loss and fragmentation of wildlife habitats caused by agricultural development in regions experiencing the greatest population growth are widely recognized as among the most serious threats to biodiversity. Thus, increasing agricultural productivity is an essential environmental goal, and one that would be much easier in a world where agricultural biotechnology is in widespread use.

Opponents of biotechnology argue that organic farming can reduce pesticide use even more than transgenic crops can. But as much as 40 percent of crop productivity in Africa and Asia and about 20 percent in the industrialized countries of North America and Europe are lost to insect pests, weeds, and plant diseases. Organic production methods would only exacerbate those crop losses. There is no way for organic farming to feed a global population expected to grow to 8 or 9 billion people without having to bring substantially more land into agricultural use.

> *Mankind has been modifying the genetic makeup of plants for thousands of years, often in ways that could have had adverse environmental impacts.*

Fortunately, many transgenic varieties that have been created specifically for use in less developed nations will soon be ready for commercialization. Examples include insect-resistant rice varieties for Asia, virus-resistant sweet potato for Africa, and virus-resistant papaya for Caribbean nations. The next generation of transgenic crops now in research labs around the world is poised to bring even further productivity improvements for the poor soils and harsh climates that are characteristic of impoverished regions.

Scientists have already identified genes for resistance to environmental stresses common in tropical nations, including tolerance to soils with high salinity and to those that are particularly acidic or alkaline. Other transgenic varieties can tolerate temporary drought conditions or extremes of heat and cold.

Ensuring worldwide food security

Biotechnology also offers hope of improving the nutritional benefits of many foods. Among the most well known is the variety called "Golden Rice," genetically enhanced with added beta carotene, which is converted to vitamin A in the human body. Another variety developed by the same research team has elevated levels of digestible iron.

The diet of more than 3 billion people worldwide includes inadequate levels of essential vitamins and minerals, such as vitamin A and iron. Deficiency in just these two micronutrients can result in severe anemia, impaired intellectual development, blindness, and even death. And even though charities and aid agencies such as the United Nations Childrens' Fund and the World Health Organization have made important strides in reducing vitamin A and iron deficiency, success has been fleeting. No permanent effective strategy has yet been devised, but Golden Rice may finally provide one.

Importantly, the Golden Rice project is a prime example of the value of extensive public sector and charitable research activities. The rice's development was funded mainly by the New York-based Rockefeller Foundation, which has promised to make the rice available to poor farmers at little or no cost. It was created by scientists at public universities in Switzerland and Germany with assistance from the Philippines-based International Rice Research Institute (IRRI) and from several multinational corporations.

Golden Rice is not the only example. Scientists at publicly funded, charitable, and corporate research centers are developing such crops as cassava, papaya, and wheat with built-in resistance to common plant viruses; rice that can more efficiently convert sunlight and carbon-dioxide for faster growth; potatoes that produce a vaccine against hepatitis B; bananas that produce a vaccine against cholera; and countless others. One lab at Tuskegee University is enhancing the level of dietary protein in sweet potatoes, a common staple crop in sub-Saharan Africa.

Admittedly, experts recognize that the problem of hunger and malnutrition is not currently caused by a global shortage of food. The primary causes of hunger in recent decades have been political unrest and corrupt governments, poor transportation and infrastructure, and, of course, poverty. All of these problems and more must be addressed if we are to ensure real, worldwide food security. But producing enough for 8 or 9 billion people will require greater yields in the regions where food is needed most, and transgenic crops are good, low-input tools for achieving this.

Transgenic crops are safe

Although the complexity of biological systems means that some promised benefits of biotechnology are many years away, the biggest threat that hungry populations currently face are restrictive policies stemming from unwarranted public fears. Although most Americans tend to support agricultural biotechnology, many Europeans and Asians have been far more cautious. Anti-biotechnology campaigners in both industrialized and less developed nations are feeding this ambivalence with scare stories that have led to the adoption of restrictive policies. Those fears are simply not supported by the scores of peer-reviewed scientific reports or the data from tens of thousands of individual field trials.

Mankind has been modifying the genetic makeup of plants for thousands of years, often in ways that could have had adverse environmental impacts and that routinely introduced entirely new genes, proteins, and other substances into the food supply. Food-grade tomatoes and potatoes are routinely bred from wild varieties that are toxic to human beings, for example. But plant breeders, biologists, and farmers have identified methods to keep potentially dangerous plants from entering the food chain.

The evidence clearly shows there is no difference between the practices necessary to ensure the safety of transgenic plants and the safety of conventional ones. In fact, because more is known about the genes that are moved in transgenic breeding methods, ensuring the safety of transgenic plants is actually easier. But the public's reticence about transgenic plants has resulted in extensive regulations that require literally thousands of individual safety tests that are often duplicative and largely unnecessary for ensuring environmental protection or consumer safety. In the end, over-cautious rules result in hyperinflated research and development costs and make it harder for poorer countries to share in the benefits of biotechnology.

Perhaps more importantly, restrictions on transgenic plants and onerous labeling requirements for biotech foods have caused many governments to block commercialization—not out of health or environmental concerns but because of a legitimate fear that important European markets could be closed to their exports. As last year's [2001] United Nations Development Report acknowledged, opposition by European consumers and very strict legal requirements in European Union member nations have held back the adoption of transgenic crops in underdeveloped nations that need them.

Furthermore, the [international treaty] Cartagena Protocol on Biosafety, adopted in January 2000, will tend to reinforce these counterproductive policies because it permits governments to erect unwarranted restrictions based on the Precautionary Principle, the notion that even hypothetical risks should be enough to keep new products off the market, regardless of their potential benefits. Thus, EU nations can restrict imports of transgenic crops from both industrialized and less developed nations, no matter how much scientific data have been presented showing them to be safe, because opponents can always hypothesize yet another novel risk.

Admittedly, advocates have to take the public's concerns more seriously. Better sharing of information and a more forthright public dialogue are necessary to explain why scientists are confident that transgenic crops are safe. No one argues that we should not proceed with caution, but needless restrictions on agricultural biotechnology could dramatically slow the pace of progress and keep important advances out of the hands of people who need them. This is the tragic side effect of unwarranted concern.

Ultimately, biotechnology is more than just a new and useful agricultural tool. It could also be a hugely important instrument of economic development in many poorer regions of the globe. By making agriculture more productive, labor and resources could be freed for use in other areas of economic growth in nations where farming currently occupies 70 or 80 percent of the population. This, in turn, would be an important step in the journey toward genuine food security. The choice is clear. Innovators must proceed with due caution. But as a report jointly published by the United Kingdom's Royal Society, the National Academies of Science from Brazil, China, India, Mexico, and the United States, and the Third World Academy of Science contends: "It is critical that the potential benefits of [transgenic] technology become available to developing countries." It is also critical that industrialized countries not stand in their way.

4

Genetically Modified Food Has Great Potential for Harm

Karen Charman

Karen Charman is an award-winning investigative journalist who writes about environmental, health, and agricultural issues.

Genetically engineered (GE) foods are bad for the environment, bad for farmers, and may not be safe to eat. These foods have been rushed to market by huge biotechnology companies. Experimental GE plants are now being grown that contain pharmaceutical drugs and even solvents, plastics, and other industrial chemicals. The pollen from these and other GE plants has contaminated some traditional and organic crops. In addition, some GE plants may contain human allergens that can sicken, or even kill, a potentially large number of people. There has been a frightening lack of research or oversight from the U.S. government concerning the human and environmental consequences of these new high-tech plants concocted in a laboratory. The government should forbid GE foods from being sold until questions about their safety are answered.

Advocates of genetically engineered food claim this revolutionary new technology is merely a more precise way to improve crops—something humans have been doing for the last 12,000 years. They don't usually acknowledge that genetic engineering gives humankind an unprecedented ability to create new life-forms by taking genes from one species and inserting them into another—something long time biotech critic Jeremy Rifkin characterizes as "a laboratory-conceived second Genesis." This is a powerful new technology and before we accept it, we must understand both its proponents' claims and the risks it poses.

The first large-scale commercial plantings of genetically modified (GM) [also referred to as genetically engineered (GE)], crops began in 1996. Although public debate and opposition to GM food has been both intense and growing throughout the world, most Americans have only begun to become aware of the issue. Nevertheless, the technology is developing quickly, and the pressures to continue using it are great. Once genetically modified organisms (GMOs)—which can grow, reproduce, mutate and migrate—are released into the environment, they cannot be removed. So before scientists and corporations remake the natural world, we would be wise to fully consider the implications GMOs raise about health and environmental safety, politics, social justice, food security and economic issues.

Questions unanswered

Agricultural biotechnology is being sold on several promises. Genetic modification of food, we are told, will enable us to save a growing world population from hunger and starvation. It will give farmers more environmentally friendly, profitable and nutritious crops to grow. Agricultural biotech will revolutionize the way we get our industrial materials, turning plants, animals and other living organisms into clean "biofactories," replacing polluting products like nonrenewable fossil fuels and synthetic chemicals.

These are all laudable goals. But whether agricultural biotechnology will achieve them or whether it will unleash greater problems than those generated by the polluting technologies it is purported to replace are questions that remain unanswered.

Four farm products—corn, soybeans, cotton and canola—currently account for nearly all of the estimated 125 million acres of biotech crops commercially grown around the world. Dairy products have also been transformed by genetic engineering; 10 percent to 30 percent of our dairy cows are injected with the controversial recombinant bovine growth hormone (rBGH) to boost milk production.

GM corn, soybeans and cotton carry genetic material from

petunias, viruses and bacteria that enable them to survive dousing with Roundup (glyphosate), the herbicide produced by biotech and chemical giant Monsanto. Other varieties of corn, canola and cotton contain genes from Bacillus thuringiensis (Bt), a natural soil bacterium that kills certain insects. Every cell of the altered plant is engineered to contain Bt, rendering the plant itself an insecticide (and it is registered as such). Other transgenic (genetically modified) crops currently approved, though not necessarily on the market, include herbicide-resistant sugar beets; virus-resistant papayas and squash; tomatoes engineered with added bacteria and virus genes to delay their ripening; Bt- and virus-resistant potatoes; soybeans and canola with altered oil content; and herbicide-resistant flax.

In the United States, unless you consciously act to avoid GM foods, you are almost certainly eating them every day. Sixty percent to 70 percent of the products on supermarket shelves contain ingredients unlabeled as being derived from GM corn, soy, canola and/or cottonseed. According to the Union of Concerned Scientists, hundreds more genetically engineered animals, plants and microbes are in the biotech industry's research pipeline. Some likely to make their way onto people's tables within the next few years include transgenic fish, chicken, rice, wheat, coffee, apples, lettuce and peanuts.

Terminator technology

The first wave of GM seeds conferred traits designed to make the crops easier for farmers to grow. The second and third waves augur something altogether different. In an attempt to offer products consumers can get excited about, nutrient levels in various foods are being genetically manipulated to boost or add vitamins, minerals and other substances thought to be healthy. The most well-known example is "Golden Rice," which has vitamin A—not normally found in rice—added.

Biotechnologists also are researching ways to introduce pharmaceutical and industrial compounds into crops. Transgenic corn and soybeans that produce veterinary vaccines and antibiotics already have been developed and grown at public agricultural research stations in the Midwest. These applications worry many farmers, since transgenic traits don't stay put once they are released into the environment, and so these compounds could end up in our food.

In an attempt to tackle this problem, the biotech sector is

busy working to create plants, that produce seeds that won't germinate, the so-called '"Terminator" technology. Biotech companies also are researching ways to genetically disable key plant functions so plants won't be able to develop normally without being sprayed with a special chemical the company also happens to sell. Such plants have been dubbed "traitor" technology, or "junkie seeds."

> *We would be wise to fully consider the implications GMOs raise about health and environmental safety, politics, social justice, food security and economic issues.*

Biotech proponents claim that transgenic Terminator plants won't spread their traits to nearby crops or related wild plants, because the Terminator plants don't produce viable seeds. The problem is, this suicidal characteristic could contaminate neighboring non-GM crops via cross-pollination. Farmers who have not elected to plant GM seeds, but who engage in the time-honored practice of saving their own seed, would be out of luck. Terminator was first developed as a way to protect biotech companies' intellectual property, and it continues to spark outrage around the world. . . .

Safe to eat?

The biotechnology industry and its promoters claim GM food is perfectly safe and has been thoroughly tested. However, the U.S. Food and Drug Administration does not require safety tests for transgenic food before it goes on the market. Instead, biotech companies have been doing their own evaluations and presenting summaries to the FDA in a "consultation process." This procedure came out of the agency's 1992 decision to regard gene-spliced food as "substantially equivalent,"—i.e., no different than food produced through conventional breeding techniques. This characterization allowed the FDA to classify transgenic food as "generally recognized as safe," which does not require pre-market safety testing.

Last year [2001] the FDA changed its tune and announced a new policy that acknowledges transgenic food is different.

The agency now requires data from biotech companies about each genetic modification, though FDA officials have not announced how they will use that information in their decision-making, says Michael Hansen, a biologist with the Consumer Policy Institute, which is part of the Consumers Union.

Meanwhile, a growing chorus of scientists are challenging the concept that GM foods are "substantially equivalent" to conventionally bred foods. According to Richard Lacey, a British medical doctor and microbiologist who specializes in food safety, genetic engineering is not only "inherently risky" but also "substantially different" from natural breeding methods, which involve sexual reproduction between the same or closely related species. With natural breeding, "every gene remains under the control of the organism's intricately balanced regulatory system," Lacey says in a deposition for a lawsuit against the FDA for releasing untested GM food into world markets. "The substances produced by the genes are those that have been within the species for a long stretch of biological time."

> *Plants won't be able to develop normally without being sprayed with a special chemical the company also happens to sell.*

With genetic engineering, biotechnologists take cells that were produced with normal reproduction methods and randomly insert foreign genetic material into them. "This always disturbs the function of the region of native DNA into which the material wedges," Lacey says. Foreign genes won't become activated in their new home by themselves, so other genes, known as promoters, must be included to try to make sure the gene functions in its new environment. These genes usually come from viruses or bacteria. "Marker" genes, which commonly are derived from a bacterial gene for antibiotic resistance, are used so biotechnologists can find the cells that received the target trait.

Lacey, who was the first to warn British authorities about the mad cow disease epidemic, says the host organism's regulatory system isn't set up to handle these foreign genes, which can cause various unpredictable imbalances that produce toxic substances or allergens, or alter the crop's nutritional value.

There also are concerns that the antibiotic-resistant bacterial genes used as markers to identify successful gene transfers will escalate the growing problem of antibiotic resistance.

The transfer of an allergen into a transgenic host has been clearly demonstrated. A transgenic soybean that contained a gene from a Brazil nut—a life-threatening allergen to some people—did cause allergic reactions, and the product was never commercialized. But gene-spliced food will contain genes from many sources that have never been part of the human diet. "Because they are not known as allergens, they can't be definitively tested for allergenicity in advance," says Jean Halloran, director of the Consumer Policy Institute. Even if potential allergens in transgenic food could be tested in advance, Lacey says, even continuous testing of transgenic food could offer only limited assurance of the product's safety.

And nothing close to that level of scrutiny over transgenic foods has taken place so far. "Peer-reviewed publications of clinical studies on the human health effects of GM food simply don't exist," and animal studies are "few and far between," says biochemist Arpad Pusztai, one of the few scientists who has actually conducted biotech food-safety tests with animals.

Independent scientists, including Pusztai and Lacey, have harshly criticized biotech industry studies as sloppy science. In a June 2001 review of transgenic food-safety studies, Pusztai writes that transgenic food is tested by comparing it with non-transgenic crops, using chemical analyses of nutrients and known toxins, which are appropriate for testing and comparing regular foods, but not thorough enough for the unpredictability inherent in GM foods. "To rely on this method is at best inadequate, and at worst, dangerous," he says.

Environmentally responsible?

Biotech proponents claim their technology will save the environment by allowing farmers to use fewer pesticides and toxic chemicals. But the evidence from transgenic crops on the market now and the mad rush by biotech companies to create GM plants that won't grow properly, or at all, unless they are sprayed with prescribed chemicals, belie that claim.

Herbicides to kill weeds in corn and soybean fields constitute the greatest use of chemicals on American farms each year, says Chuck Benbrook, director of the Northwest Science and Policy Center in Sandpoint, Idaho. The main use of GM technology so far has been to engineer herbicide-resistant corn and soybeans, which enable farmers to simplify their weed management by spraying broad-spectrum weed killers throughout the growing season. Between 1997 and 2000, the average amount of pesticides increased with transgenic herbicide-resistant crops, USDA data reveals. Insecticide use did decrease dramatically with the use of Bt cotton, but Benbrook says the reduction is likely temporary.

> *By the summer of 2000, virtually all of the tested organic corn samples from the Midwest showed some degree of transgenic contamination.*

Relying on chemical sprays to manage pests, weeds and diseases is a silver-bullet approach that creates a pesticide treadmill. Drawing on 50 years of toxic chemical use to control cotton pests, Benbrook says every family of chemicals had about a decade before their targeted pests became immune. "There is no reason to expect that resistance will take much longer to emerge in regions where Bt crops are planted extensively," he wrote in the October 2001 issue of *Pesticide Outlook*. He also predicts increases in herbicide use, especially with the popular Roundup-ready crops, as weeds develop resistance to the chemicals. . . .

Contaminating native plants

Last fall's [2001] announcement of the transgenic contamination of native corn plants in Oaxaca, Mexico, an ancestral homeland for corn, also has raised alarms about how fast GMOs can spread. Crop homelands need to be preserved, because that's where scientists go to look for traits to overcome catastrophic pests or diseases, as was necessary in 1970 when the Southern corn leaf blight wiped out 15 percent of the U.S. corn harvest. The GMO contamination occurred despite Mexico's 1998 ban on planting transgenic corn and may have resulted from seeds that sprouted after falling off government trucks, which brought bioengineered corn into Oaxaca as food aid.

Concerns about wandering transgenic traits are taking on new urgency with the development of gene-spliced pharmaceutical and industrial plants. According to the USDA's Animal and Plant Health Inspection Services (APHIS), the primary government agency regulating field trials of bioengineered plants, 30 sites are now testing GM crops in the environment. The identity of the compounds is considered "confidential business information" and cannot be released. But there are reports that some of the substances already growing in GM-plant field tests include antibiotics, vaccines, plastics, fuels and solvents.

APHIS science adviser Sally McCammon says the combination of buffer zones, sowing the crops at different times to vary when they shed pollen, and planting extra barrier crops around both the test crops and adjacent fields should ensure the transgenes don't escape into food crops growing nearby. But Hansen questions whether stringent controls for transgenic industrial or pharmaceutical crops are always followed. Since even basic information about the field trials is not available, he says it is impossible to know.

The National Academy of Sciences found serious flaws in APHIS's regulation of biotech field trials. Under current rules, a company can simply inform APHIS what it wants to grow to obtain permission. Such field tests are performed under "notification"—actual environmental impact assessments have been virtually nonexistent. And the vast majority of transgenic field tests—96 percent in the year 2000—are conducted under these rules.

What the transgenic compound is intended for determines how it is regulated; currently there are no rules specifically governing industrial transgenic plants, though the U.S. Environmental Protection Agency says it plans to implement some. "At present, as long as your intent is not to use it for a pharmaceutical purpose—it can be a research chemical or an industrial solvent—you can put it into the plants, do a simple notification to APHIS with virtually no data, and then you can commercialize it, as was done with avidin-producing corn. Even the National Academy of Sciences noted this was a glaring loophole that needs to be closed," Hansen says.

Good for farmers?

Unyielding consumer opposition to GMOs around the world has severely limited export markets for U.S. corn and soybeans. As a result, farmers have had to deal with both substantial drops in price and newly created competition from foreign farmers who are filling the demand for non-GM corn and soybeans, says Dan MacGuire, agricultural policy analyst with the American Corn Growers Association. Since farmers are already struggling with historically low commodity prices that fall below their costs of production, this is a hit they can ill afford.

> *The biotech industry and its supporters have always maintained that labeling would somehow stigmatize the product and have fought bitterly to prohibit it.*

One of the only bright spots for farmers over the last decade has been organic farming. What started out as a small niche market for health- and environment-conscious consumers has turned into a $9 billion industry, with sales growing at least 20 percent a year for the past 10 years. But organic farmers are starting to lose their lucrative markets—and consumers are losing their ability to choose non-GM food—because GM traits are turning up in organic crops. By the summer of 2000, virtually all of the tested organic corn samples from the Midwest showed some degree of transgenic contamination, says Fred Kirschenmann, director of the Leopold Center for Sustainable Agriculture at Iowa State University. GM contamination has destroyed the small but promising Canadian organic canola market, and Janet Jacobson, president of the Northern Plains Sustainable Agriculture Society, says she doesn't know any organic farmers who can assure the purity of their organically grown corn, soybeans or canola.

Eden Foods, a company that produces a wide range of organic foods, including Edensoy organic soy milk, recently announced efforts to create a sustainable supply of nonbioengineered organic corn for its products. The effort, which is modeled on their system for procuring organic soybeans, involves close collaboration with seed suppliers, 100 organic corn growers, and malting and milling companies. Each follows specific protocols to guarantee that the corn is protected from transgenic contamination. These steps are documented, and the corn is tested every step of the way. "This process—the paperwork, the storage of the corn samples so that we can duplicate any tests we do, and the storage of the tests themselves—

is more difficult, time-consuming and costly than everything we do to certify that our products are organic," says Eden chairman and president Michael Potter. Besides requiring nearly two sets of full-time staff, making sure their corn is GMO-free has doubled the cost of the corn and increased their malt costs by 24 percent. . . .

A just and democratic technology?

Crop diversity is already threatened by our modern industrial farming system that plants a relatively small number of varieties across millions of acres. Biotech patents will further erode any remaining crop diversity, making both farmers and the public more dependent on agribusiness corporations like Monsanto and DuPont that produce genetically engineered seeds.

Civil society groups around the world are challenging corporate claims on life patents. Activists from more than 50 countries are pressing for a treaty that would establish the Earth's gene pool as a global commons. More than 300 organizations have signed onto the effort and are now working to enshrine the treaty in legislation around the globe.

Because of the many questions surrounding genetically modified food, in January 2001 more than 130 nations signed the Biosafety Protocol, a treaty that, among other things, would give countries the right to refuse imports of GMOs if they believe the shipments would harm their environment. The U.S. government opposes this concept, known as the Precautionary Principle, and tries to dispute it at every international forum possible.

With the strength of the U.S. government behind the biotech industry, unindustrialized nations and civil society groups are finding it difficult to secure careful evaluation and regulation of bioengineered food. Still, the battle seems far from over.

Consumers overseas and increasing numbers of consumers here in the United States are adamant that at the very least, GM food should be labeled as such. But the biotech industry and its supporters have always maintained that labeling would somehow stigmatize the product and have fought bitterly to prohibit it. Despite intense lobbying by probiotech forces, the European Union recently took steps to strengthen labeling requirements for food containing GMOs and began labeling animal feeds.

Clearly, enormous health, environmental and social issues are emerging as genetically engineered foods move into the marketplace. Norman C. Ellstrand, a geneticist at the University of California, Riverside, who studies how genes are transferred between domesticated and wild plants, advises us to proceed thoughtfully and cautiously with genetic engineering. "Creating something just because we are now able to do so is an inadequate reason for embracing a technology," he wrote in the April 2001 issue of *Plant Physiology*. "If we have advanced tools for creating novel agricultural products, we should use the advanced knowledge from ecology and population genetics, as well as social sciences and humanities, to make mindful choices about how to create the products that are best for humans and our environment."

Considering that GMOs, once released, cannot be recalled to the lab, and given the many thorny questions this radical technology raises, Ellstrand's advice that we be mindful is only prudent.

5

An Epidemic of Mad Cow Disease in the United States Is Inevitable

Christine Wenc

Christine Wenc has a doctorate in environmental history and the history of medicine and is the former editor of the Stranger, *a Seattle weekly.*

In the past several decades, deadly new pathogens called prions have been found in the beef supply. Prions can cause bovine spongiform encephalopathy (BSE), commonly known as mad cow disease. BSE can spread to humans, killing those who eat the meat of the infected animals. When a cow infected with BSE was found in Washington State in December 2003, the U.S. government quickly assured consumers that this was an isolated incident and there was no danger to the meat supply. In reality, BSE can be easily spread as a result of the methods used by modern meat processing plants where one infected cow can spread the disease to thousands of others. Unless these huge plants change the way that they kill and process cattle, an epidemic of mad cow disease is inevitable in the United States.

We all know (or should know) that factory meat farming is violent and environmentally destructive. You don't have to be a vegan activist to be disturbed by the conditions in which most meat animals live and die. And you probably already know

Christine Wenc, "Cannibal Cows & Dying Deer," *The Stranger*, August 27, 2003. Reproduced by permission of the author.

that a large percentage of pesticide use, water pollution, and groundwater depletion is caused by the intensive cultivation of grain used to feed livestock, especially cattle. The environmental damage caused by the cattle themselves—the enormous expanses of land required, the destruction of native vegetation, the problem of what to do with all that poop—has fundamentally altered entire ecosystems. So that every supermarket can be packed with cheap beef and milk, every town can have scores of fast-food chain restaurants, and most Americans can comfort-. ably participate in the fallacy that a meal is not a meal unless it contains meat, we feed, pump full of drugs, and confine about 96 million cattle every year. We kill about 30 million.

We would all be better off without so much meat. Still, the cattle industry has proved as resilient as most Americans are oblivious to the process by which that burger came to their table. Despite a decade's worth of bad news about beef, the average American still eats 66 pounds [in 1999], and beef consumption typically goes way, way up in the summer months. How many hamburgers have you had since Memorial Day?

A new player, however, has emerged in this game and could force the issue and destroy the multibillion-dollar beef industry: the infective prion, the agent that causes mad cow and similar diseases. Unfortunately, prions also have the potential to cause human suffering on an enormous scale. The recent discovery of mad cow disease in Canada [and Washington in December 2003] and a good look at the ineffectual efforts to avoid it . . . show that the disease is not far away from us at all.

Meat market prions

Until the 20th century, most people who ate meat either grew or hunted it themselves; the animals you ate lived where you did and ate what they had evolved to eat. Now, though, we have the factory meat industry, to which it is difficult to offer any compliments. From the near-extermination of American buffalo to the return of the low-paying, dangerous slaughterhouse job to the present treatment of living creatures as commercial products packed in tight boxes and fed everything from cardboard to chicken shit, its unsavory history goes back more than 100 years.

But the meat industry may yet be undone—not by squads of vegetarian activists, but by itself. All evidence suggests that the power of the infective prion has been fortified and widely spread in the past 30 years by the practices of the factory meat farm. No simple cousins of the E. coli bacteria, prions apparently have their own biological category, are undetectable by ordinary tests, and resist all normal methods of disinfection. They cause fatal degenerative brain diseases that have no treatment and no cure, cross species barriers, and have killed more than 130 people in the U.K. [United Kingdom] who ate infected beef, and there is a possibility that many more will die. If anything is going to bring down factory meat farming, the prion is it.

Unfortunately, if this happens, it may also bring down anyone who's been exposed to meat or animal-derived products in the last 30 or 40 years—that is, for all practical purposes, everyone. Vegetarians and vegans are not immune; prions may exist in the bovine materials used in common vaccines. Did you chew on Altoids mints in the 1980s? They used to be made with beef gelatin. Had surgery? Prions survive standard medical autoclaving disinfection procedures, and prion disease has been spread from human to human via contaminated equipment. If a slaughterhouse processes one cow infected with mad cow disease, the meat of those that follow may become infected too, making even organic beef suspect. And many cosmetics and other pharmaceuticals contain bovine products.

There is some good news in prion research: It seems that tetracycline antibiotics may slow the incubation period, so that it might, say, take you 15 years to develop symptoms rather than 10. Of course, since there is currently no way to diagnose prion disease until symptoms appear, this may be less useful than it sounds. There's also evidence that part of the population may be genetically resistant.

Still, it does seem that anyone who's devoted enough time to the subject is definitely not casual about the possibilities, especially when the woefully inadequate United States Department of Agriculture (USDA) and Food and Drug Administration (FDA) efforts to prevent American mad cow disease are considered. Canada's rules were similar to ours. . . .

"Unusual disease agents"

What is a prion anyway? The word "prion" (pronounced "pree-on") was coined by Nobel Prize–winner Stanley Prusiner for the agent that causes transmissible spongiform encephalopathies, also known as TSEs (be ready for many more acronyms). A combination of the words "infective" and "protein," "prion" is a word that Prusiner apparently made up partly for its media-friendly sound. Probably the most famous TSE is bovine spongiform encephalopathy (BSE), or mad cow disease, which showed up in England in 1986. A close second might be kuru, also known as the cannibalism disease. There is also a naturally occurring prion disease in humans called Creutzfeldt-Jakob disease (CJD), which researchers say spontaneously arises in one in a million people; animal versions apparently appear at the same rate. However, like much of the research done with TSEs, this rate is basically an educated guess. . . . When BSE spread to people in England during the 1980s and 1990s from eating infected beef, the human version was called Variant Creutzfeldt-Jakob disease, or vCJD. It differs from regular CJD in a number of ways, but perhaps the most significant is that it strikes the young; British teenagers have died of vCJD, whereas regular CJD is a rare disease of the elderly. However, there is evidence that some cases of Alzheimer's disease are actually incidents of misdiagnosed CJD.

> *In the United States, dogs are eating dogs, pigs are eating pigs, and until very recently, cows were eating cows.*

Prions are highly unusual disease agents, and researchers admit that we don't know much about them. We do know that prions are most densely concentrated in the brain and central nervous system, but they are also found in muscle tissue; depending on the species, prion disease can be spread through eating infected tissue. . . . But an infective prion is not an organism; it has no DNA. Yet, somehow, it still manages to infect a host and reproduce itself, which places it outside most known biology; as one researcher put it, prions "differ from all known microorganisms and viruses." The most widely accepted theory is that infective prions are mutated versions of the normal proteins found mostly in the brain. The mutant prions—which seem to have the same chemical formula but a different structure than nonmutant proteins—somehow join the normal ones and cause them to fold themselves into the mutant structure. This then spreads throughout the brain and causes spongiform encephalopathy; the brain becomes a mass of spongy holes.

Loss of motor control and dementia set in, and in humans, the patient dies in about six months to a year. An infected host shows no immune response; there currently is no way to definitively test human beings and most animals for prions until the subject is dead and a brain biopsy is performed.

Turning animal wastes into products

Though prions may have always existed, it is clear that human activity has fortified and multiplied them in ways that would not have happened without the factory farm. Rendering, "turning animal wastes into marketable products," as John Stauber and Sheldon Rampton put in their [1997] book *Mad Cow, U.S.A.* was the crucial element in the dissemination of the BSE prion. The rather disturbing but extremely common practice of feeding cattle, as a protein supplement, meat and bone meal (MBM) made up of rendered animal bodies (including the meat and bones of cows—only about half of a cow can be used for food) went on in England and the United States for decades. In the U.S., a modified version of the practice, which is held directly responsible for the spread of BSE in Britain, still exists on a wide scale.

In England, after the first case of BSE was reported in 1986, more than 180,000 English cows contracted the disease—far more than official projections. British researchers discovered that a cow had to eat only one gram of infected cow tissue—a piece the size of a peppercorn—to be infected. If it is rendered and made into feed, one infected cow can infect thousands of others.

Rendering has a long history—think soap made from beef tallow—but 20th-century industrial agriculture took the process to a whole new level. Animal bodies are dumped into huge vats and cooked down to create, as one byproduct, MBM; it looks like cornmeal. This includes not only millions of leftover farm animal parts but also road kill and the remains of hundreds of thousands of cats and dogs euthanized by animal shelters. So in the United States, dogs are eating dogs, pigs are eating pigs, and until very recently, cows were eating cows. According to Stauber and Rampton, four billion pounds of rendered animal goes into animal feed every year. If you have eaten nonorganic beef in the past 30 years, you have eaten the meat of cannibal cows.

Why are cattle fed this stuff anyway? For one, something

has to be done with the remains of millions of cattle slaughtered here every year. For another, cows fed protein supplements produce more milk and grow to a larger size in a much shorter period of time, and MBM protein is cheaper than soy. Dairy cows, most of which are now pumped up on productivity-enhancing drugs, must be fed high-protein supplements. Giving a cow bovine growth hormone, or BGH, requires that you also give it MBM; retired dairy cows become hamburger themselves, and, making a neat circle, their unused body parts are rendered into MBM again.

> *Meat processing plants . . . use mechanical 'advanced meat recovery systems' designed to get the very last bits of meat off a carcass, including the head; this goes into hamburger and processed meats.*

In 1997, years after it was clear what was causing the spread of BSE in Britain, the FDA finally banned the feeding of protein supplements derived from cows to cattle in the United States. Canada's feed ban took effect the same year. Nevertheless, cattle-derived feed is still widely available; according to FDA regulations it must only be clearly labeled with the warning "not to be fed to ruminant animals," like cows, sheep, and deer, and feed mills must store it separately. Whether or not farmers follow these directions is up to them. Also, pigs, dogs, and cats can still be fed cattle MBM, and when these animals die, they can be fed to cows. This is why recent research on the way prions can cross the species barrier—and the fact that animals infected with a TSE do not necessarily show symptoms—is so disturbing. Even more disturbing is the fact that the body of the Canadian mad cow, which was not originally suspected of having BSE, was rendered, joined with the bodies of thousands of others and made into animal food shipped to the U.S. and elsewhere.

[In the summer of 2002] at a national conference for wildlife professionals in Denver focusing on the deer and elk TSE known as chronic wasting disease (CWD), Rick Race, a researcher with the National Institutes of Health, asked a very important question: "What's happening in animals that don't get sick?" His team injected mouse brains with a large dose of a hamster TSE. After a few years, a few of the mice got sick and died of prion disease, but most did not. Then the "healthy" mice were killed and their brain tissue was injected into new mice. The entire second group of mice contracted a fatal TSE. A new strain of the hamster prion disease had been created, one that was particularly deadly to mice. Race's research shows that even though the infective prion can exist in a host without causing disease, this does not diminish its infectivity should that host's nonsymptomatic body become a means of transmitting the agent.

So if an apparently healthy animal is killed, rendered, and fed to other animals, not only might the apparently healthy animal be carrying a TSE, but the TSE may then cross the species barrier to infect and sicken a new animal. Granted, these experiments used intracerebral inoculation to transmit the infective prions, a method far more effective in transmitting TSEs than eating infected tissue or having contact with it. Still, they demonstrate something very disturbing, something to which government officials and meat-industry executives in this country have been extremely slow to respond.

BSE in the USA

In November 2001, the Harvard Center for Risk Analysis (HCRA) published a report analyzing the risk of BSE occurring in the United States. The group reached the conclusion that "there is little chance that the disease will be a serious threat either to the American cattle herd or to public health." Why? Because even if BSE were introduced into the American cattle population, "in all cases, the disease fails to take hold and dies out, usually within a matter of a few years." According to the press release, HCRA's computer modeling showed that even in the worst-case scenarios, the number of sick animals would remain small, and the amount of contaminated meat entering the human food supply and causing vCJD would be "minute."

It is very important, however, to understand the essential condition for Harvard's conclusion to be truly reassuring. That condition is the enforcement of the 1997 FDA ban on feeding cattle-derived meat and bone meal to cattle.

Despite the feed ban, compliance and enforcement among renderers and feed mills have been less than rigorous. When the GAO, the Congressional General Accounting Office, looked into the matter for a report issued [in 2002], it found that the

FDA's enforcement of the feed ban was limited, and the inspection data was "significantly" flawed. Their report noted that there are no penalties for violating the feed ban and that the FDA has no enforcement strategy for feed-ban compliance.

The FDA's database is also filled with serious problems; for instance, entries for about 45 percent of all inspections lack the information that would connect them with an individual feed mill or renderer—crucial if a BSE case were to be traced—and 438 entries did not mention whether prohibited proteins were included in cattle feed, the point of the whole ban in the first place. The GAO wrote, "Even if the FDA were to actively enforce the feed ban, its inspection database is so severely flawed that— until corrected—it should not be used to assess compliance." Last summer [2002] the FDA website's most recent "update" on the BSE situation was dated June 2001, and it revealed that 22 percent of all feed mills and renderers inspected that handled the forbidden proteins were in violation of the feed ban.

Then there is the predictable (and, in my opinion, irresponsible) response of the Cattlemen's Beef Association, the marketing arm of the cattle industry. Their official media statement on the Canadian situation lists six reasons why BSE is not a problem here, all of which I consider misleading and manipulative. For instance: "BSE affects older cattle. . . . The vast majority of cattle going to market in the U.S. are less than 24 months old." "The surveillance system targets all cattle with any signs of neurological disorder." "The U.S. banned imports of cattle and bovine products from countries with BSE beginning in 1989." "The BSE agent is not found in meat. It is found in central nervous system tissue such as brain and spinal cord."

Okay. The reason BSE "affects older cattle" is that usually only older cattle live long enough to show visible signs of BSE. A cow younger than 24 months could easily be infected, and therefore be infective, without showing symptoms. If our surveillance system targets only cattle with obvious signs of disease, we are still potentially missing many animals with BSE. And banning imports does nothing about our domestic situation.

And let's take a long look at that last misleading statement "The BSE agent is not found in meat. It is found in central nervous system tissue such as brain and spinal cord." True, prions are found in the highest concentrations in central nervous system tissue rather than in muscle. But cattle spinal cord and brain tissue are still allowed to enter our food supply, usually in processed meat like hot dogs. Beef stock and beef flavoring are made by boiling skeletons, including the spinal column. The USDA has opted not to tell consumers if the meat products they are buying might contain these tissues, because "labeling and warning statements should be reserved for known hazards, which BSE is not in the United States." Meat processing plants also still use mechanical "advanced meat recovery systems" designed to get the very last bits of meat off a carcass, including the head; this goes into hamburger and processed meats. And the bolt-gun method used to kill meat cattle has been shown to splatter brains all over the rest of the carcass. In any case, recent research shows more clearly than ever that prions are found in muscle tissues—in meat.

> *It is absurd to think that wanting food free of fatal disease agents, from animals that did not spend their lives being tortured, makes you into some kind of hippie freak.*

The Cattlemen also mention the Harvard study, the one that argued the risk of BSE in the United States was low provided the feeding-cows-to-cows ban was being enforced. The three-year, $500,000 Harvard study was funded by the USDA, it should be pointed out, which is quite friendly with the American cattle industry; many upper-level USDA officials were formerly executives in the meat business and vice versa. George Gray, director of the Harvard study, says the study was peer reviewed and that new regulations have been proposed for industry because of it. "Our task was to characterize the state of U.S. BSE risk management. Testing of cattle does nothing to increase protection against the disease." This is arguable—in the U.K., BSE has been nearly eliminated, largely due to intensive testing of even healthy-looking cattle, as well as enforcement of a much more severe feed ban. The rules are similar in Europe. In the Old World, cows no longer eat meat. (To be fair, the USDA and the FDA—most likely in response to the GAO report, not the Harvard report—have started to take action. Never fear. Advance notices of proposed rulemaking on the people-eating-cattle-brains problem are scheduled to begin soon!)

There are additional problems with the Harvard study: It looked only at the effects of introducing between one and 500

BSE-infected cattle into the country. But we have imported millions of cattle from Canada, and as author John Stauber told me, we don't know if there is one mad cow there or a thousand. We also import cattle from Mexico, where our feed-ban labels are written in English. The Harvard study also focused on the possibility of BSE being introduced into the United States, not on the possibility that it might already be here unreported. But given the long incubation period for TSEs, as well as the fact that testing actual American cows for the disease did not start until 1990, it is quite possible that we have our own strain of BSE. Though bans on British beef and cattle went into effect almost immediately when BSE was first found in the U.K., we lived in the identical meat processing situation as the Brits for decades, on a much wider scale. Stauber says the Harvard study is "garbage."

Is it possible that the USDA is deliberately not testing as much as it should? The USDA performs important marketing work for the multibillion-dollar American beef industry. If even one case of BSE were made public, it would likely be decimated, much as the English industry was and as the Canadian probably will be.

Finally, the USDA tells us that our BSE testing "vastly exceeds international standards." This statement is pure bunk. Between 1994 and 2001, the USDA tested only 4,870 cattle brains for BSE—.0005 percent of our 96 million cows. The USDA now announces that it has "tripled" the number of BSE tests, to 20,000 in the past year. But between 2001 and 2003, England—a country dwarfed by our western cattle-raising states—tested more than 500,000 cows. In Japan, where BSE was found a few years ago, all cattle are tested. Stanley Prusiner says that U.S. testing standards are "appalling." I believe it is safer to eat beef in the U.K. than it is here.

Pushing the status quo

Conservatives and corporate interests have put a lot of energy into creating the impression that wanting something other than the status quo—a status quo that is increasingly dangerous to public health—is akin to being communist. But it is absurd to think that wanting food free of fatal disease agents, from animals that did not spend their lives being tortured, makes you into some kind of hippie freak. It's partly our own fault for being ignorant and complacent; we have spent a long time accustomed to cheap food, too long uncurious about where it comes from and indifferent to the suffering our habits have created for other creatures. Should a BSE disaster come to pass, I can't help but consider that we are simply reaping what we have sown. Our environmental problems may come to include the effects of biological agents not previously known—or, in the case of genetic engineering, not previously in existence.

6

Mad Cow Disease Is Not a Threat to the United States

Elizabeth Whelan

Elizabeth Whelan is president of the American Council on Science and Health.

When mad cow disease was discovered in December 2003 in a cow in Washington State, millions of consumers became concerned about the safety of their meat. Despite the dire warnings of cattle industry critics, the American meat supply is safe. The U.S. Department of Agriculture was able to prevent the spread of the disease beyond a single case. Moreover, the odds of anyone contracting mad cow disease are extremely small. People face much greater risks driving to work or school every day than they do from eating beef. It is in the interest of the beef industry to closely monitor itself to ensure that mad cow disease does not become a problem.

When tests on a cow slaughtered [in December 2003] near Yakima, Washington, tested positive . . . for what is known in lay terms as "Mad Cow Disease," consumers were understandably bewildered and anxious. What did this mean for their food selection and health?

Is it safe to eat beef? Is the USDA falling down on the job and allowing an infectious agent into our food supply?

Is it possible that this one infected cow transmitted the disease to many more? Is there anything I can personally do to ensure the beef I purchase and prepare is safe? If the beef is as safe

Elizabeth Whelan, "The Mad Cow Kerfuffle," *New York Sun*, December 26, 2003.

as USDA Commissioner Ann Veneman keeps telling us, why are countries such as Japan and Korea now refusing to import American beef? Is this just another food scare du jour with absolutely no basis in scientific fact??

There are many questions and at this point, only a few answers:

First, Mad Cow Disease is a nickname for bovine spongiform encephalopathy [BSE], a transmissible, slowly progressive, degenerative fatal disease affecting the central nervous system of cattle. It is a member of a group of similar diseases that have been found in other animals like sheep. BSE only affects cattle. There is, however, a disease similar to BSE called Creutzfeldt-Jakob Disease, a serious, life-threatening neurological disorder that occurs in human beings.

CJD occurs at a rate of about 1 in 1 million worldwide, and is not associated with consumption of beef. After an outbreak of BSE in Britain in the 1980s, a new type of CJD was diagnosed in a small number of people there and was named "variant CJD," or "vCJD." These cases occurred in people who consumed beef that may have been contaminated. There is both epidemiological and laboratory evidence that the agent that causes BSE in cows causes vCJD in people.

Given these facts, the risk of Mad Cow Disease as a threat to human health is not merely a theoretical threat, as is the case with human exposure to trace levels of chemicals that at high doses cause cancer in lab animals. However, as we will see, the current risk to Americans eating beef, while not theoretical, is exceedingly small.

Monitoring safety and quality

Second, the fact that the USDA was able to pick up this presumptive case of BSE in a single cow is testimony to the sensitivity and efficacy of our agricultural surveillance system. Indeed these reports are good news reassurance that we have a system in place to monitor the safety and quality of our beef supply.

Third, contrary to what has been erroneously harped upon in the press, Mad Cow Disease, while it is an infectious disease, is not transmitted from one living animal to another. It is not like Foot and Mouth Disease, which is a highly communicable, infectious disease. Indeed the primary way a cow becomes infected with BSE is by eating feed that has been contaminated with parts of brain and spinal cord tissue from other infected animals. (By some unknown mechanism, animals can also develop the disease spontaneously.)

Fourth, even if you were to eat beef from an infected cow itself a highly unlikely scenario you would almost definitely not be exposed to the "prions," the aberrant proteins that are the causative agents of BSE. This is because BSE does not show up in the muscle and thus cuts of beef such as steak, roasts, and chops have virtually no risk.

> *The fact that the USDA was able to pick up this presumptive case of BSE in a single cow is testimony to the sensitivity and efficacy of our agricultural surveillance system.*

There is a theoretical risk of BSE contamination of ground beef if the beef in processing gets mixed with specks of neural tissue but this risk is infinitesimally small. Thus, the calls from food-nanny groups such as the Nader-inspired Center for Science in the Public Interest to avoid pizza toppings, taco fillings, hot dogs, and salami, are scientifically without merit in other words, baloney.

Fifth, the mere fact that certain countries initially announce their intention to ban American beef imports means nothing scientifically. Such a move is a normal part of ongoing trade wars between countries plus it represents a public relations move for the leadership of a country that wishes to communicate to the public that they are doing their job "protecting" them even though no risk exists. (The U.S. did the same thing temporarily banning Canadian beef imports earlier this year [2003] when a single case was identified in Canada.)

Along similar lines, any beef scare brings out advocates with agendas other than public health, including vegetarians and animal rights groups who take advantage of a scare to generally discourage people from eating virtually any animal product.

Sixth, food is a highly emotionally charged issue. When it comes to scares, to paraphrase an old proverb, reports of exaggerated risks can be halfway around the world before the truth gets its boots on.

The key here is to make our own decisions based on science, not fear.

The bottom line: There is no reason whatsoever to hesitate to eat American beef. Like the rest of the American food supply, our beef supply is safe. If we only spent as much time focusing on real, significant risks (for example, cigarette smoking, skipping our influenza vaccine, overexposure to sunlight etc.) as we do to a minuscule risk like BSE in beef, our nation would be even healthier than we are today.

7

Organic Food Is Expensive, Bad for the Environment, and Potentially Deadly

Alex Knapp

Alex Knapp is a staff writer for Tech News, *the student newspaper of Worcester Polytechnic Institute.*

Advocates of organic farming tout the safety and nutritional superiority of foods grown without synthetic pesticides or chemical fertilizers. However, organic fruits, vegetables, and meats are little different from other foods, except that they cost considerably more than their nonorganic counterparts. The manure used to fertilize organic fields can contain deadly *E. coli* bacteria, which on occasion is transferred to consumers who eat the produce. Furthermore, studies have shown that organic foods do not contain larger quantities of nutrients, vitamins, or minerals than other foods. Consumers should think twice about paying extra for organic food.

Organic foods are a burgeoning industry in the United States. Although they encompass only about 3% of the total agricultural market in the US, that number is rapidly growing. Organic foods are those that are produced without the use of synthetic chemicals or through genetic engineering. They are also substantially more expensive than conventional foods. It is the opinion of many Americans that organic food is healthier and safer than conventional foods; an opinion that the organic food industry strives to cultivate. However, as former Agriculture Secretary Dan Glickman pointed out, "The organic label is a marketing tool. It is not a statement about food safety."

> *The organic label is a marketing tool. It is not a statement about food safety.*

One major misconception about the organic food industry is that their products are not grown using pesticides. This is not entirely accurate. It is true that organic producers do not use any synthetic pesticides. However, they use many "organic" pesticides, which are pesticides derived from natural products. As Alex Avery of the Center For Global Food Issues points out, "Organic pesticides are the most heavily used agricultural pesticides in the U.S." Pesticides used by organic farmers account for over 25% of the total pesticide use in the United States. This figure does not include the most commonly used organic pesticide, [naturally occurring soil bacterium] Bt [*Bacillus thuringiensis*], because it cannot be measured in pounds per active chemical use. Also, many other common organic pesticides are not included in this figure because they are not measured, either.

Effects of organic pest control

Two of the most common organic pesticides, copper and sulfur, are used as fungicides by organic growers. Because they are not as effective as their synthetic counterparts, they are applied at significantly higher rates. This is disturbing because both sulfur and copper have greater environmental toxicity than their synthetic counterparts. The two most commonly used insecticides by organic farmers are Bt and oil (usually petroleum or soybean oil). However, a substantial amount of oil has to be used to achieve the same results as synthetic insecticides. Other organic pesticides are generally extracted from plants. One such pesticide, pyrethrum, has a demand satisfied by the hand harvest of about 600 million flowers per year. This accounts for a significant amount of green space that could otherwise be used as wildlife preserve or to grow food.

One type of pesticide that organic growers admittedly do

not use, in any form, are herbicides. However, the development of herbicides has led to low-till farming methods that significantly decrease soil erosion and increase the sustainability of agricultural land. Bereft of this option, organic growers must rely on methods that lead to increased soil erosion, unless they maintain a strict crop rotation schedule.

> **" The extra bucks that you're shelling out don't provide an extra dime of safety or nutrition. "**

Another type of pest control used by organic growers is so-called "biocontrol" techniques. This type of pest control relies on insects, fungi, or bacteria to destroy pests that are harmful to crops. Organic farmers promote this as a less environmentally damaging method of pest control. However, the introduction of such biocontrol can have a debilitating effect on local ecosystems. Since most biocontrol organisms are not native to the areas in which they are employed, they have led to substantial ecological devastation in several areas.

Organics not healthier

Not only do organic farmers make the claim that their products are environmentally safe, they also claim that organic products are healthier. However, there is no evidence that this is the case. As a *U.S. News & World Report* article stated, "organic foods are no richer than other varieties in vitamins, antioxidants, and other nutrients. In addition, organic produce causes an increased risk of food poisoning. According to the CDC [Centers for Disease Control and Prevention], in 1996, the last year for which data is available, 36% of people suffering from E. coli 0157:H7 infection contracted it from organic food. This strain of E. coli is particularly vicious—it kills thousands of people every year, and can cause substantial damage to the liver or kidneys. Organic foods are susceptible to E. coli infection because manure and compost are commonly used fertilizers in organic farming, and both often contain large amounts of the bacteria. In response to the claim of E. coli infection, Whole Foods Market, Inc., an organic producer, issued a statement that composting should eliminate the risk of infection. However, composting is generally performed at 130° to 140°, but temperatures of 160° are necessary in order to kill this E. coli strain.

Although organic farms make the claim that their products are better for the environment, produce less toxic chemicals, and are safer and healthier, the facts do not seem to bear these claims out. Although it is true that there are potential long-term health threats stemming from the use of synthetic fertilizers, the evidence for such a threat has yet to be substantiated in the nearly 40 years since this danger was first identified in Rachel Carson's [book] *Silent Spring*. However, the risks of using organic foods are known and substantiated. This is not to say that organic foods are substantially unsafe—feel free to eat organic. Just be aware that the extra bucks that you're shelling out don't provide an extra dime of safety or nutrition.

8

More Americans Are Choosing Organic Food for Safety and Health

Richard McGill Murphy

Richard McGill Murphy is a journalist who has written for the Wall Street Journal, *the* New Republic, *and the* New York Times Sunday Magazine.

Those concerned with the safety, quality, and purity of their foods are turning to organically farmed products in growing numbers. An increasing fear of tainted food has created a surging demand for fruits, vegetables, and meats raised without pesticides, hormones, additives, and genetically modified organisms. When mad cow disease was discovered in a cow in Yakima, Washington, in December 2003, demand for organic beef surged. Despite reassurances from the U.S. Department of Agriculture about the safety of conventionally grown food, every year more and more consumers are choosing to buy organic food.

Two days before this past Christmas [2003], Oregon cattle rancher Doc Hatfield was sitting in his office after finishing his outside chores, when the phone rang. A customer, worried about catching the human equivalent of mad cow disease from eating Hatfield's beef, wanted to know what steps he had taken to protect his animals.

The 65-year-old Hatfield was perplexed, but he calmly explained to her that mad cow disease spreads when cows eat feed mixed with boiled-down slaughterhouse byproducts. Hatfield's

High Desert Ranch cows, on the other hand, are fed a diet of grass and natural grain that contains no hormones, antibiotics or other artificial additives. "Nothing is a thousand percent," Hatfield assured her. "But we're as safe as you can get."

Hatfield didn't understand the woman's sudden interest in bovine spongiform encephalopathy (BSE), a disease that had wreaked havoc on the British beef industry in the late 1980s and early '90s. Then he turned on his television. On the evening news, U.S. Secretary of Agriculture Ann Veneman was announcing that federal food inspectors had discovered the first suspected case of BSE in the U.S. in neighboring Washington state.

The incident, so far, has turned out to be a single, isolated case. As is the tendency when food safety scares occur, shocks of alarm pulsed through consumerdom and the media in the immediate aftermath of the disclosure. Government health and safety officials, lobbyists, agencies and corporate affairs representatives sprang into action. They responded decisively and methodically to consumers' fears and questions as the nation momentarily curbed its huge appetite for beef. But only momentarily. . . .

Consumers demanding information

December 23, 2003, may well pass into food safety annals as little more than a footnote. Americans' consumption of about $900 billion in fresh and processed foods each year—through channels such as supermarkets, corner delis, price clubs and mass merchants, convenience stores, restaurants, hospitality and other food service providers, as well as other conduits—won't be likely to change a lick as a result of this lone incident.

What is changing, though, is a broader context of consumerism within which the mad cow scare took place. The challenge for those vested and invested in the food business is that more and more ordinary people are becoming more demanding about everything they buy. They want to know precisely what's in what they buy. What are the ingredients? What was the manufacturing process? Who made it? How was it made? Where? Were the conditions safe? Humane? What impact did the manufacture of the item have on the environment, and the people in the environment? People are asking these questions and demanding "transparency" and forthrightness in answers to them.

For the American food business, the telephone call to Doc Hatfield on the afternoon of Dec. 23rd told of a story behind the headlines, illustrative of an American consumer public that has begun to behave differently—more information-hungry, more active, more discriminating—in an environment where food safety crises crop up in America and around the world. Crisis public relations may have been sufficient to quell concerns about America's food supply this time round, but food manufacturers, distributors and retailers may not be so fortunate in the future.

> *Mainstream urbanites want to know where their food is coming from.*

In the weeks that followed that first late-December phone call, Hatfield had at least 50 calls and e-mails from prospective customers interested in buying his natural beef because of concerns over BSE. However, Hatfield, who heads Oregon Country Beef, a family ranch cooperative, says consumer demand had been increasing even before the latest scare. Oregon Country Beef saw same-store sales of its meat jump 43 percent in the last quarter of 2003. Sales for the year reached $18 million, 24 percent higher than in 2002. The cooperative's biggest customers include the Whole Foods Markets natural food chain and a number of high-end independent grocery stores in the Pacific Northwest.

"When we started 18 years ago, our customers ranged from hippies to urban gourmets," says Hatfield, who founded the business with his wife Connie. "But now mainstream urbanites want to know where their food is coming from. It's not just about nuts and twigs any more."

Not just granola

Hatfield's right. It's not just "nuts and twigs" who are buying food produced without chemicals, hormones and other additives. As more Americans make health, nutrition and food safety a higher priority, they're buying more organic and natural food. "Organic" is one of the labeling terms in the food business Americans equate most closely with transparency, and so they're driving high double-digit sales growth in food categories that are generally flat year-on-year. Americans bought $13.5 billion worth of natural and organic food in 2002, 8.9 percent more than they did a year earlier, according to the latest data provided by SPINS, a San Francisco market research company that tracks retail sales scanned at supermarkets, natural food stores, mass merchandisers and drug stores. Of that, organic food sales were $8.2 billion, or 17.8 percent higher than in 2001. SPINS estimates that natural and organic food and beverage sales rose more than 12 percent. That rate of growth is considerably higher by a ratio of 4-to-1 than that of conventional grocery product sales.

In an exclusive poll for American Demographics conducted in mid-January [2004] by Harris Interactive, a polling firm in Rochester, N.Y., of 2,289 respondents, 1 person in 4 was either "extremely concerned" or "very concerned" about the safety of meat and produce. Almost 2 in 5 Americans (39 percent) believe organic or natural foods are healthier. And 1 in 3 believes they are safer.

"The Baby Boomers are driving demand for organic food in

> **More than half of Americans . . . have tried organic food.**

general, because they're health-conscious and can afford to pay higher prices," says Professor Steven G. Sapp, a sociologist at Iowa State University who studies consumer food behavior. More than half of Americans (54 percent) have tried organic food, according to a survey for Whole Foods Market conducted by Synovate in August 2003. In the American Demographics' survey, 28 percent of respondents say that they buy more organic or natural foods than they did five years ago. And 31 percent would like a greater assortment of organic and natural food in their local supermarket.

Consumers are also putting more organic and natural products in their shopping carts because they want more information about how their food is produced. Food can only be labeled organic if it meets the USDA's [U.S. Department of Agriculture's] strict standards: no pesticides, no hormones, no genetically modified organisms (GMOs) and no artificial additives of any kind. . . .

Touting organics' virtues

No sooner had the sick Holstein in Washington been destroyed than a broad array of interest groups started using the scare to push their own agendas. Led by People for the Ethical Treatment of Animals, animal rights activists announced that the outbreak was yet another good reason for Americans to go vegetarian. Organic food advocates saw an opportunity to tout the virtues of an organic diet, pointing out that no organically raised cow had ever been diagnosed with mad cow disease.

"The BSE scare is a great opportunity for organic producers to explain what organic beef is," says Katherine DiMotta, executive director of the Organic Trade Association. "Many consumers didn't understand that you could have an organic cow."

The Center for Consumer Freedom, a nonprofit advocacy organization funded by food companies and the restaurant industry, responded with aggressive attack ads that dismissed the vegetarians and the organic community as alarmist, self-serving hypocrites who sought to deny Americans their God-given right to eat whatever the heck they wanted. The National Cattlemen's Beef Association, which has an annual budget of nearly $68 million, of which $7.45 million is spent on government lobbying, seized on the fact that the sick cow had been found as proof that the USDA's cattle inspection system worked perfectly.

Beef industry critics dismissed these claims, pointing out that inspectors see only a tiny fraction of the 30 million cows that are slaughtered each year and arguing that the USDA was a wholly owned subsidiary of U.S. corporate agriculture in general and Big Beef in particular. After all, [USDA] Secretary [Ann] Veneman and 11 of her senior aides had previously worked as beef industry lobbyists, they pointed out. . . .

Organic goes corporate

Organic food sales are still quite small, accounting for no more than 3 percent of the U.S. food market, according to the Organic Consumers Association. But while conventional food sales have been essentially flat in recent years, organic food has been racking up steady double-digit increases every year since 1991. That's despite the fact that organic products are usually 30 percent to 50 percent more expensive. "If you plot out that graph, in 20 years most food sold at U.S. grocery stores will be organic," says [executive director of the Organic Consumers Association Ronnie] Cummins.

A far-fetched scenario, perhaps, but as consumers' demand grows, major food companies are entering a sector that was once the domain of small farmers. In 1999, General Mills, the $11.5-billion food behemoth whose brands include Betty Crocker, Hamburger Helper and Green Giant vegetables, bought Small Planet Foods, maker of Cascadian Farm and Muir Glen, the country's largest processor of organic tomatoes. And in January [2004], Borden and Land O' Lakes' parent Dean Foods Co., with $9.5 billion in sales, bought Horizon Organic Dairy for $216 million in cash and assumed the milk producer's $40 million debt.

However, big food producers avoid giving consumers the impression that their organic products are healthier than their conventional offerings. H.J. Heinz Co., for example, launched its own organic ketchup brand in 2002, says spokesman Robin Teets. Although industry-wide organic ketchup sales have doubled in the past two years to $6 million from $3 million, that's still a tiny percentage of the $500 million U.S. ketchup market. "We don't position any organic product as being healthier nutritionally than any other product," Teets says. "Instead, we treat organic food like any other market niche. Basically, it's a lifestyle choice."

Inspired by the success of Whole Foods and Wild Oats Natural Marketplace, Safeway, Kroger and other mainstream grocery chains now offer organic food under their own private labels. Even the world's largest retailer, Wal-Mart Stores Inc., which caters to middle America, stocks organic food on its shelves. According to SPINS, more than 75 percent of all natural products—food, beverages, beauty aids and health supplements—are now sold in supermarkets, drug stores and mass merchandisers.

Where's the beef?

The beef industry is no exception to this trend. Mel Coleman, Jr., is a fifth-generation Colorado rancher who heads Coleman's Natural Beef in Denver, one of the nation's largest producers of natural beef. Coleman used to sell most of his meat to natural food stores, but that's changed in recent years. Today, mainstream supermarkets account for 60 percent of total sales, Coleman says.

Like Oregon Country Beef, Coleman beef comes from cattle raised without growth hormones or so-called sub-therapeutic antibiotics both commonly used in the mass-market beef industry. In 2003, Coleman's sales shot up 38 percent, compared with a 2 percent to 3 percent increase for conventional beef. Sales spiked after the mad cow disease report: For the week ending January 16 [2004], orders were up 25 percent to 30 percent over the previous week. "There's been a whole lifestyle change as compared to years past," Coleman says. . . .

> *Food can only be labeled organic if it meets the USDA's strict standards: no pesticides, no hormones, no genetically modified organisms . . . and no artificial additives of any kind.*

During her December 23 [2003] TV appearance, Secretary Veneman announced that U.S. beef was perfectly safe and that she herself planned to eat beef for Christmas. Even so, more than 40 countries moved to ban U.S. beef imports, including Japan, the biggest overseas consumer. The $30-billion beef industry normally sells around 10 percent of its product abroad. Suddenly, the industry was looking at $2 billion in lost 2004 export revenues, according to Chris Hurt, an agricultural economist at Purdue University.

Surveys showed that Americans intended to eat less red meat. On January 16 [2004], a *Wall Street Journal*/Harris Interactive poll found that 1 in 5 Americans (21 percent) planned to change their eating habits out of fear of mad cow disease. Most (78 percent) said they would eat less beef, while 16 percent said they would stop eating beef altogether. By late January, consumers were once again eating beef.

After the news of mad cow disease in the U.S., the National Cattlemen's Beef Association's polls showed consumers had a high level of awareness and concern about mad cow disease peaking at 96 percent at the end of December, but almost equally high levels of confidence in the safety of U.S. beef. By mid-January, 90 percent of respondents were confident that U.S. beef was safe, up 2 percentage points from a previous poll taken in September.

"Most people are comfortable with U.S. meat," said Dr. Christine Bruhn, a food safety expert who runs the Center for Food Research at the University of California-Davis. "Some aren't comfortable, and those people are either switching away from meat or looking for meat raised in a different way."

However, if more mad cow cases turn up, the U.S. organic beef industry could see a truly dramatic spike in demand. Alternatively, American consumers could start getting their protein from chicken, pork or soybeans. No matter what happens, though, we can be sure that all sides of the debate will continue to articulate their views at top volume.

Meanwhile, Doc Hatfield and his fellow organic and natural meat producers are enjoying the attention and increased sales that have come their way. "BSE has accelerated an already growing trend of people wanting to know where their food comes from," Hatfield says.

9

Irradiated Food Can Cause Cancer and Other Health Problems

Public Citizen

Public Citizen is a national, nonprofit consumer advocacy organization that lobbies for health, safety, and environmental protections.

It is well known that exposing food to radioactive materials can kill dangerous pathogens such as *Salmonella* and *E. coli*. However, foods treated in this manner are unsafe for human consumption. Food irradiation has been linked to rare cancers, genetic mutations, and other deadly conditions in both laboratory animals and human beings. The irony is that irradiation would be unnecessary in most cases if foods were not tainted with fecal matter and other preventable forms of contamination during storage and processing. The FDA and other government agencies have consistently lied about the safety of food irradiation. Consumers should stay away from these dangerous foods unless they are willing to pay with their health.

The scientific community is in agreement that food irradiation is among the most thoroughly researched technologies of the 20th century. Where there is no agreement, however, is whether "treating" foods with high doses of ionizing radiation to kill pathogens and extend shelf-life poses health risks to the people who eat these products.

Food irradiation research began in 1921, when a U.S. Department of Agriculture scientist discovered that X-rays killed the *Trichinella spiralis* bacteria commonly found in pork. Two years later, the results of the first animal feeding studies to evaluate the safety and wholesomeness of irradiated foods were published.

In the 80 years since, dozens of foods—bananas, ground pork, onion powder, papayas, beef stew, potatoes, clams, chicken, apricots and many others—have been irradiated and fed to numerous types of animals, mainly rats, mice, dogs, monkeys and hamsters.

At least six experiments involving people—including one involving children—have been conducted.

Virtually every biological assessment of test subjects has been made: animal fetuses have been dissected, biopsies have been taken, DNA and chromosomes have been examined, red and white blood cells have been counted, enzyme levels have been measured, and so on.

Over these eight decades, dozens of studies have drawn into question the safety and wholesomeness of irradiated foods. A wide range of health problems have been observed in animals—and, in a few cases, people—who ate irradiated foods.

Substantial health problems

Whether the food was "treated" with gamma rays, X-rays or near-speed-of-light electrons, many adverse health effects have been observed, including but not limited to premature death, mutations and other genetic damage, fetal death and other reproductive problems, residual radioactivity, immune system dysfunction, fatal internal bleeding, a rare form of cancer, organ damage, blood disorders, tumors, nutritional deficiencies and stunted growth.

Here are some noteworthy examples:

• A chromosome abnormality called polyploidy—which has been associated with leukemia and direct exposure to radiation—was detected in children who ate recently irradiated wheat.

• Polyploidy and a blood disorder were detected in men and women who ate a diet containing a variety of irradiated foods; and elevated red blood cell counts were detected in men and women who ate irradiated potatoes.

• The carcinogenesis process was promoted in rats fed a chemical called cyclobutanones, which are formed in certain irradiated foods, and which do not occur naturally in any food.

• "Considerable amounts of radioactivity" were detected in the liver, kidney, stomach, gastrointestinal tract and blood serum of rats fed irradiated sugar [according to researcher A.K. De].

• Rats fed irradiated beef died from internal bleeding; others fed irradiated beef suffered "general incoordination, spastic hopping gait and sometimes complete loss of movement with dragging hindquarters. Those most severely affected often became completely prostrated a short time before death" [as C.E. Poling writes].

• In U.S. Army tests, more dogs and rat pups died, and dogs gained less weight than those fed unirradiated foods; and a rare form of cancer developed in rats.

• Rats fed a variety of irradiated foods gave birth to more dead offspring.

• Mice fed recently irradiated food led to embryonic and fetal deaths, and shorter lifespans.

• Fruit flies grown in an irradiated medium were born with a variety of mutations.

Additionally, human blood cells exposed to irradiated food components have undergone genetic damage, including "grossly damaged" chromosomes and [according to P.C. Kesavan and M.S. Swarminathan] "considerable inhibition of mitosis and chromosome fragmentation."

Many researchers who have observed health problems in animals that ate irradiated foods have said that these problems could not be attributed to consuming irradiated foods. Instead, researchers have often made unsubstantiated claims that these health problems were due to dietary factors or experimental anomalies.

> **"** *A wide range of health problems have been observed in animals—and, in a few cases, people—who ate irradiated foods.* **"**

In many other cases, researchers who documented health problems in their raw data simply failed to discuss these problems in the summaries and conclusions of their reports. Abnormalities in reproductive performance, blood counts, enzyme levels, organ function, weight gain and other measurements have been recorded, only to be ignored in summaries and conclusions. . . .

By downplaying and ignoring raw data suggesting that irradiated foods may not be safe for human consumption, scientists from a wide variety of universities, institutes, organizations and agencies have deprived government officials, the food industry, food scientists and, ultimately, the American people of the complete picture of the potential health problems associated with these products.

> *Many chemicals known or suspected to cause cancer and birth defects, and chemicals that can damage the central nervous system, have been detected in irradiated foods.*

By misrepresenting raw data, these scientists have ignored seemingly minor health problems that, in the long term, could result in more serious effects—particularly if multiple problems work in combination, or if problems fester unnoticed for months or years. . . .

Toxic chemical compounds

Furthermore, irradiation results in the formation of dozens of chemical compounds, many of which have toxic properties. The scientific record of these chemicals goes back 50 years. During this time, many chemicals known or suspected to cause cancer and birth defects, and chemicals that can damage the central nervous system, have been detected in irradiated foods. Among these are benzene, toluene, methyl ethyl ketone, octane, acetone, ethanol, hexane, heptane and pentane. "Safe" levels for these chemicals in irradiated foods have yet to be determined.

Recently, chemical byproducts formed in irradiated foods called cyclobutanones (or 2-ACBs) were shown to promote the carcinogenesis process in rats, and to cause genetic damage in rats and in human cells. Cyclobutanones have never been found to occur naturally in any food.

These findings, coming in four consecutive experiments since 1989, contributed to the European Union's decision in

Dec. 2002 against expanding irradiation for several additional types of food, including shrimp, cereal flakes and frog legs. The findings have also delayed a proposal by the Codex Alimentarius Commission—which sets food-safety standard for more than 160 nations—to allow any food to be irradiated at any dose, no matter how high.

In conclusion, the researchers wrote:

> [S]ince our results point toward toxic, genotoxic and even tumor promoting activity of certain 2-ACBs, we strongly recommend to carry out further research, including confirmation of our results by other laboratories, to elucidate a possible risk associated with the consumption of irradiated fat-containing foods. . . . Numerous questions still remain to be answered, and much research is left to be done, before a qualified risk assessment can be performed.

These findings are particularly disturbing, given that 2-ACBs have been found in numerous foods that contain fat, including beef, chicken, pork, eggs, cheese, fresh- and salt-water fish, salmon, shrimp, mangoes and papayas. The types of fat from which 2-ACBs derive—such as oleic, palmitic and stearic acids—are contained in nearly all foods.

In one study, researchers found 2-ACBs in chicken that was irradiated 13 years earlier. 2-ACBs are so easily detected and can be formed at such low radiation doses that they are often used as chemical "markers" to determine whether food has been irradiated. The European Union, for example, has officially adopted this technique to determine whether fat-containing foods have been irradiated.

FDA, U.S. Army and other federal officials have consistently misled Congress about the potential hazards of food irradiation.

In addition to concerns related to 2-ACBs, many other warnings have been issued by researchers during the past 50 years.

Among them:

• "An increase in concentration of a mutagen in food by irradiation will increase the incidence of cancer. . . . It will take four to six decades to demonstrate a statistically significant increase in cancer due to mutagens introduced into food by irradiation. . . . When food irradiation is finally prohibited, several decades worth of people with increase cancer incidence will be in the pipeline" [according to G.L. Tritsch]. . . .

Flawed approval process

Despite a vast body of evidence that irradiated foods may not be safe for human consumption, and despite numerous warnings from researchers, food irradiation has been endorsed by the World Health Organization (WHO), the United Nations' Food and Agriculture Organization (FAO), the International Atomic Energy Agency (IAEA) and the Codex Alimentarius Commission. And, the process has been legalized in more than 50 countries.

In particular, the WHO has played a role in abandoning the original research agenda it co-drafted in 1961, which urged experiments into whether irradiated foods are toxic or radioactive; whether they could cause cancer, mutations or nutritional deficiencies; and whether the scientific expertise even existed to answer these fundamental questions.

The process by which the U.S. Food and Drug Administration (FDA) has legalized food irradiation has also been flawed. The FDA has legalized irradiation for several major classes of food—including fruit, vegetables, pork, chicken, beef and eggs—despite numerous shortcomings:

• Since 1983, FDA agency officials have knowingly and systematically ignored federal regulations and their own testing protocols that must be followed before irradiated foods can legally be approved for human consumption.

• Since 1986, FDA officials have legalized irradiation for major classes of food while relying on nearly 80 studies that the agency's own expert scientists had dismissed as "deficient." (The FDA legalized the irradiation of eggs in July 2000, for instance, based on three "deficient" studies, one of which was conducted in 1959.)

• None of the seven key studies that FDA officials used to legitimize their first major approval of food irradiation in 1986 met modern standards. (One of them had actually been declared "deficient" by FDA toxicologists; three others had never been translated into English.)

• FDA officials have systematically dismissed evidence suggesting that irradiated food can be toxic and induce genetic damage. Much of this evidence resulted from government-funded research submitted to the FDA and members of Congress as early as 1968.

• FDA, U.S. Army and other federal officials have consistently misled Congress about the potential hazards of food irradiation, and about the reasons that past research initiatives have failed to demonstrate that irradiated food is safe for human consumption.

International objections

Following a rapid expansion of food irradiation in the U.S., the European Parliament [EP] voted in December 2002 against expanding the list of foods that could be irradiated in the 15-nation European Union, pending additional scientific evidence regarding the safety of irradiated foods. Shrimp, frog legs, cereal flakes and several other foods were proposed for addition to the current list, which is limited to spices and seasonings. The EP went so far as to reject a proposal to collaborate with the WHO on research into the safety of irradiated foods.

Further, the EU—citing concerns over 2-ACBs—formally opposed a Codex proposal to remove its 10 kGy[1] maximum dose and allow any food to be irradiated at any dose, no matter how high. France, Germany, Japan, the Netherlands, Poland, Sweden, South Korea and the United Kingdom also opposed the proposal. Under this pressure, a key Codex panel in December 2002 abandoned the proposal.

The decision is significant, to say the least: Codex sets food-safety standards on behalf of more than 160 countries representing more than 90 percent of the world's population. And, Codex standards are enforceable under World Trade Organization (WTO) rules. . . .

In retrospect, the 40-plus-year history of analyzing the safety and wholesomeness has been compromised to the extent that a complete reassessment is required in order to protect Americans, as well as millions of people throughout the world where food irradiation is legal, from health risks. This reassessment should take the form of published, peer-reviewed research in the areas of toxicology, food science, radiation

1. A kGy, or kilogray, is a unit of measurement for radiation.

chemistry, nutrition and other relevant fields.

Taken together, the well-documented health hazards of ir-radiated foods; the flawed processes by which food irradiation has been legalized and endorsed by U.S. and international agencies; the recent caution exhibited by the European Union and the Codex Alimentarius Commission; and the myriad un-answered questions related to this technology, make any pro-posal to legalize or endorse additional types of food for irradia-tion, to expand use of irradiation, or to broaden the production and distribution of irradiated foods is ill-advised.

10

Irradiation Makes the Food Supply Safer

Robin Brett Parnes, William C. Idell, Audrey L. Anastasia Kanik, and Alice H. Lichtenstein

The authors are journalists who write on science and food issues for national publications, including Nutrition Today.

Food-borne illness can easily be prevented with food irradiation. By exposing food to small doses of radioactivity, food processors prevent thousands of people from being exposed to *Salmonella, E. coli*, and other pathogens. In addition to saving lives, food irradiation is also useful for killing insects, extending the shelf life of perishable foods, and delaying the ripening of fruits and vegetables. Irradiation ensures a safer, more abundant food supply for people throughout the world.

Food-borne illness is a major source of preventable morbidity and mortality. The Centers for Disease Control and Prevention (CDC) estimates that in 1999 food-borne illness caused 76 million illnesses, 325,000 hospitalizations, and 5,200 deaths in the United States. Between 1990 and 1999, nearly 300 outbreaks of food-borne illness occurred in schools, affecting approximately 16,000 children. Among all illnesses attributable to food-borne transmission, 30% are caused by bacteria, 67% by viruses, and 3% by parasites. Of the deaths attributable to food-borne illness, bacteria accounted for 72%, parasites 21%, and viruses 7%. Six pathogens have been identified as being responsible for more than 90% of the estimated food-related deaths: Salmo-

Robin Brett Parnes, William C. Idell, Audrey L. Anastasia Kanik, and Alice H. Lichtenstein, "Food Irradiation: An Overlooked Opportunity for Food Safety and Preservation," *Nutrition Today*, vol. 38, September/October 2003, pp. 174–85. Copyright © 2003 by Lippincott/Williams & Wilkins. Reproduced by permission.

nella (31%), Listeria (28%), Toxoplasma (21%), Norwalk-like viruses (7%), Campylobacter (5%), and Escherichia coli 0157:H7 (3%). Overall, the federal government spends approximately $1 billion on food safety measures. In addition, the Economic Research Service (ERS) of the US Department of Agriculture (USDA) estimates that through incurred medical costs, productivity losses, and premature deaths, food-borne illness costs the United States between $7 billion and $37 billion per year.

Irradiation reduces risks

More than 50 years of research have demonstrated that irradiating food can safely and effectively reduce illness from food-borne pathogens. It can also extend the shelf life of foods by delaying ripening, inhibiting spoilage, and minimizing contamination. To a large extent, these potential benefits have yet to be realized in the United States because of the slow acceptance of this technology.

> *More than 50 years of research have demonstrated that irradiating food can safely and effectively reduce illness from food-borne pathogens.*

The food industry has been reluctant to sell irradiated foods because of a perception that consumers are unwilling to buy products associated with radiation. Unfortunately, little hard data are available to gauge potential consumer acceptance in the 21st century. Nevertheless, to date, 52 countries have given approval for irradiation of more than 100 food products.

Food irradiation uses ionizing radiation to extend the shelf life and increase the safety of several foods. Ionizing radiation is a form of electromagnetic radiation that contains adequate energy to dislodge electrons from the electron cloud surrounding individual atoms and molecules. The removal of electrons creates highly charged reactive products known as ions. The sources of ionizing radiation used in food irradiation are gamma rays, X-rays, and high-energy electron beams. . . .

The use of gamma rays for food irradiation uses manmade radioactive substances that emit high-energy gamma rays as they revert back to a more stable energy state . . . making it extremely expensive at this time. . . .

Killing salmonella, mold, and E. coli

An estimated hundreds of millions of people worldwide suffer from diseases caused by consuming contaminated food. Food irradiation can be used to effectively eliminate pathogens that cause food-borne illness. For example, doses between 1 kGy[1] and 3 kGy reduce or eliminate populations of food-borne pathogens on produce. Additionally, 3 kGy dose can kill 99.9% of salmonella in poultry and an even higher percentage of E. coli in ground beef. One approach to interrupt the reproductive mechanism of the pathogenic microorganisms is to disrupt their DNA. The larger the organism, the smaller the doses of irradiation. . . . Irradiation is not recommended to control viruses or toxins, because [of] their extremely small DNA. . . .

Food irradiation can also be used to extend the shelf life and decrease losses resulting from spoilage of fresh fruits and vegetables, as well as meats, fish, and poultry. The ERS reports that, although it is not possible to determine an exact number, evidence suggests that losses of edible food (primarily from microbial growth and the presence of insects and mold) on the farm, as well as between the farm and retail levels, can be "significant for certain commodities.". . .

Inhibition of sprouting

For many plant foods, inhibition of sprouting resulting from irradiation can increase their storage life. A radiation dose of up to 0.15 kGy can inhibit the sprouting of tubers, such as potatoes, yams, onions, garlic, and ginger, by inhibiting cell division within the food.

Insect disinfestation

Contamination by insects is a problem with dried grains, cereals, coffee beans, and dried fruits, as well as fresh citrus fruits, mangoes, and papayas. Most insects can be rendered sterile with radiation doses between 0.05 kGy and 0.75 kGy. It has been suggested that imported fresh fruits and vegetables be

1. A kGy, or kilogray, is a unit of measure for radiation.

treated with a dose of 0.15 kGy as a quarantine measure to help control for fruit flies.

Decontamination

Irradiation is a viable approach to treat spices, seasonings, fruits, and vegetables that can become heavily contaminated by pests because of poor environmental and processing conditions. The lack of heat in irradiation can preserve the flavor, color, and aromas of these products while effectively decreasing the microbial load. Spice can be irradiated at doses up to 30 kGy.

Delay ripening

Doses of 0.25 kGy to 0.35 kGy can suppress the ripening of bananas, mangoes, papayas, guava, and other tropical and subtropical fruits. Food irradiation causes little change in the "fresh" characteristics of foods, because the process does not raise the temperature of foods much, if at all, at the doses used.

Sterilization

Sterilization of foods can be achieved at doses of 10 kGY to 50 kGy. If packaged adequately, foods that are sterilized by irradiation can be stored for years without refrigeration, similar to canned (heat-sterilized) foods. Sterilized food is useful in hospitals for patients with severely impaired immune systems, such as patients with AIDS or patients undergoing chemotherapy. Sterilized irradiated foods are also currently being used at the International Space Station.

Environmental advantages

Food irradiation could replace chemical fumigants and use of vapor heat processes, resulting in a reduction or elimination of chemical residues in food and less harm to the environment.

Nutritional consequences

The lack of any substantial effect of irradiation on the nutritive value of food has been confirmed by several scientific organizations throughout the world. The Joint Expert Committee on the Wholesomeness of Irradiated Food, formed by the United Nations' Food and Agriculture Organization (FAO), the International Atomic Energy Agency (IAEA), and the World Health Organization (WHO), evaluated available data on irradiation and the nutrient content of foods in 1964, 1969, 1976, and 1980 and concluded that irradiation up to 10 kGy "introduced no special nutritional or microbiological problems." The Advisory Committee on Irradiated and Novel Foods in the United Kingdom reaffirmed this point in 1986, as did the Scientific Committee on Food of the Commission of the European Community the following year. The American Dietetic Association states in its position paper on food irradiation, "food irradiation offers negligible loss of nutrients or sensory qualities in food as it does not substantially raise the temperature of the food during processing."

Safe to eat

Since the 1950s, hundreds of research groups have examined possible toxicologic effects of consuming irradiated foods. The studies have been performed on a variety of animals, including rats, mice, dogs, monkeys, hamsters, and pigs and humans, by researchers throughout the world, examining potential physiologic effects using a range of radiation doses. No adverse effect of consuming irradiated food has been reported.

> *An estimated hundreds of millions of people worldwide suffer from diseases caused by consuming contaminated food.*

In 1980, along with its finding about the effects of radiation on the nutritive value of foods, the Joint Expert Committee stated that "the irradiation of any food commodity" up to an overall average absorbed dose of 10 kGy "presents no toxicological hazard" and requires no further testing. In 1982, the FDA performed a systematic review of 400 studies. The agency ranked the studies based on several factors that determined their statistical significance and the power of their findings. The FDA concluded that there are no compounds identified that constitute a toxicologic risk in the amounts in which they would occur when a food is irradiated at doses up to 1 kGy. Although some of the studies reported adverse effects, none were corroborated. In 1994, an expert committee of WHO followed up on the evaluation of studies done before 1980. Looking at more than 500 studies, the committee reiterated the earlier findings that food irradiation causes no toxicologic, microbiologic, or nutritional changes that adversely affect human health. Then in 1999, a Joint FAO/IAEA/WHO Study Group assessed the safety and nutritional adequacy of food irradiated to doses above 10 kGy. After a thorough review, the Study Group concluded that irradiated foods using several sources under a variety of conditions are toxicologically safe for human consumption.

Environmental concerns

Concerns have been expressed regarding the safety of the storage and transport of the materials used to irradiate food. This is not an issue for facilities that use electron-beam and X-ray technologies, because these systems do not use any radioactive materials. Because the cobalt-60 has a half-life of 5.3 years, a source must be periodically refreshed by adding "pencils." When the energy of cobalt-60 "pencils" is no longer at a useful operational level, it is either recycled or discarded. Canisters, developed according to standards set by the IAEA, have been designed to ship radioactive material. Handling procedures for cobalt-60 must conform to the strict regulatory procedures established by the Department of Transportation (DOT), the Environmental Protection Agency (EPA), and the Nuclear Regulatory Commission (NRC). Cobalt-60 poses a minimal threat to the environment because of its short half-life and physical form, a solid metal.

Worker safety

The NRC has established strict controls to protect the safety of workers in irradiation plants. Plants are built with several safety checks, including layers of redundant protective systems to detect equipment malfunctions and a maze of thick concrete walls designed to prevent workers from being exposed to ionizing radiation. Potentially hazardous areas are continuously monitored, and, when products are being irradiated, a system of interlocks prevents unauthorized entry. In the more than 30 years that these facilities have been in operation, there have been no major accidents associated with food irradiation that endangered either public health or environmental safety. . . .

> *No adverse effect of consuming irradiated food has been reported.*

Because irradiation can potentially affect the characteristics of a food product in a way that is not obvious to a consumer, all irradiated food sold in the United States is required by the FDA and USDA to be clearly labeled with the international irradiation symbol, the Radura and the words, "treated by irradiation" or "treated with radiation." However, currently, since the passage of the most recent Farm Bill [in 2002] the federal government is considering allowing the use of an alternative term, such as "cold pasteurized" to indicate that a product has been irradiated. Additional statements may be included by the manufacturer to inform the consumer why the food has been irradiated (eg, "to eliminate harmful bacteria" or "to control spoilage") or how to store the food to best maintain its quality—provided they are truthful and not misleading. If irradiated ingredients (eg, spices) are added to foods that have not been irradiated, the FDA does not require special labeling on such retail packages, because it is obvious that such foods have been processed. However, FSIS [Food Safety and Inspection Service] regulations require that irradiated meat and poultry ingredients in multi-ingredient meat and poultry products be identified on the list of ingredients. Special labeling is also required for foods not yet in the retail market that may undergo further processing to ensure that foods are not irradiated multiple times. Labeling is not required for food served in restaurants. . . .

Foods granted approval for irradiation

Since passage of the Food Additives Amendment, the FDA and USDA have approved the use of irradiation for several food products, including wheat, potatoes, pork, spices, various fruits and vegetables, poultry, and red meat.

Although evidence indicates that irradiation is safe and effective and is endorsed worldwide by prominent scientific and health-related organizations, availability of irradiated food products in the United States has been limited. According to a report by the General Accounting Office (GAO) that was published in August 2000, an estimated 97 million pounds of food products are irradiated in the United States every year, which is only a small portion of the total amount of food consumed. Spices, herbs, and seasonings comprise the majority (98%) of food products that are irradiated. It has been speculated that food processors and retailers have kept the supply of irradiated foods low because they perceive that consumers are reluctant to buy irradiated foods and because of the high capital costs of irradiation equipment. As a result, healthcare and food service establishments, serving customers who are at risk of food-borne disease, remain the primary users of irradiated food.

Why is food irradiation controversial?

Despite its numerous benefits, the food industry has been hesitant to fully use food irradiation technology because of perceived misgivings consumers have about radiation in general. Additionally, retail outlets carry only a limited number of irradiated products, because they fear negative attention from the few vocal public interest groups (namely, Public Citizen, Cancer Prevention Coalition, and Food and Water, Inc) opposed to food irradiation, who claim that it is used to mask unsanitary slaughtering and processing practices. However, food irradiation does not replace, but rather complements, proper food handling by producers and processors. Meat and poultry establishments that use irradiation are required to meet sanitation and Hazard Analysis and Critical Control Point (HACCP) regulations. For the most part, consumers do not fully understand and have not thought much about food irradiation as a processing or food safety technology. Moreover, consumers trust our food supply and are willing to purchase irradiated foods. In fact, the few studies of consumer attitudes toward food irradiation that have been conducted show that, given information about the technology, half or more will choose irradiated foods. In a survey conducted in November 2001, 52% of the respondents said that because of the threat of bioterrorism, the government should require irradiation to help ensure a safe food supply.

The recently passed 2002 Farm Bill includes a provision directing the Secretary of Health and Human Services (HHS) to redefine pasteurization to include any process that HHS has approved to improve food safety. Irradiation is one of those processes. Consequently, companies may be able to use "cold pasteurized" or "electronic pasteurized" on products that have been irradiated, which, if implemented, could potentially allay consumer concerns about food irradiation. The Farm Bill also allows for schools participating in the school lunch program to purchase irradiated meat for students by the end of the year.

Although the US food supply is considered to be among the safest in the world, food-borne illness remains a serious public health problem. Increased use of food irradiation could provide an additional tool with which to reduce the occurrence of food-borne illness and costs associated with such outbreaks. Furthermore, it can increase the availability of a wider variety of foods to the consumer by extending shelf life of highly perishable foods. Theoretically, an initial capital investment to increase food irradiation capacity in the United States could be offset by decreased loss resulting from spoilage. Critical in this process would be adequate consumer education and strong government oversight. Regardless of changes that may be made to labeling requirements, food irradiation is an underused technology that could potentially play a major role within a comprehensive strategy to keep our food supply safe.

11

Pesticides in Foods Are Poisoning Consumers

Charles M. Benbrook

Charles M. Benbrook is the president of Benbrook Consultant Services in Sandpoint, Idaho. He worked on agricultural, science and regulatory issues in Washington, D.C., from 1979 through 1997, and served as the agricultural staff expert on the Council for Environmental Quality during the Carter administration.

Recent tests have shown that pesticides in food can cause health problems for consumers, especially children and infants. Even trace amounts of pesticides in foods such as apples, grapes, tomatoes, and strawberries have been shown to cause brain and liver damage in young children. While the U.S. Department of Agriculture continues to insist that organic food is no healthier than conventionally grown produce, children who are fed organic food have been shown to have much lower pesticide levels in their bodies. Scientists will continue to argue over how much pesticide is dangerous, but consumers wishing to protect their children should avoid foods that have been sprayed with pesticides.

O ver the last two decades the organic community has had a love-hate relationship with food safety issues in general, and pesticide risks in particular. For the most part, the community has chosen to not prominently feature food safety as a reason to "buy organic," and instead has focused messages targeting consumers on freshness and taste, and the environmental and soil quality benefits of organic farming systems and technologies.

Charles M. Benbrook, "Why Food Safety Will Continue Driving Growth in Demand for Organic Food," address at EcoFarm Conference, Monterey, CA, January 24, 2003. Reproduced by permission of the author.

Anti-pesticide activists have not shown the restraint evident across the organic food industry. They have embraced organic farming as the surest way to reduce pesticide use and risks. The message is getting through. A majority of consumers in virtually all surveys voice significant concerns over pesticides in food. In "The Packer's" *2003 Fresh Trends* survey, 63 percent of shoppers buying organic food stated a preference for "fewer chemicals in food" and 51 percent said organic food is "Better for me/my family." The next most frequently cited reason—"Better for the environment"—was identified by 37 percent of those surveyed.

For reasons beyond the control of the organic community, there is now a raging food safety, food quality debate underway around the world. It is focusing on the impacts of different farming systems and technologies—conventional farming versus biotech versus IPM[1] versus organic. The . . . recent . . . [negative] PR from conventional ag interests shows how low those threatened by the success of organic farming will go in trying to shake consumer confidence in organic food. Hopefully the organic community now realizes that the industry's critics must not be allowed to set the tone and drive the direction of this very important debate.

> *63 percent of shoppers buying organic food stated a preference for 'fewer chemicals in food' and 51 percent said organic food is 'Better for me/my family.'*

Activists opposing genetic engineering (GE) around the world have been criticized in the media as paranoid and anti-progress. Some have stumbled when asked ". . . well, if GE is not the answer, how would you solve today's food production and food security challenges?" With increasing frequency, activists point to organic farming as the more desirable technological path. Proponents of biotech have not been bashful in responding.

This debate is long overdue, important, and ultimately,

1. IPM (integrated pest management) is a combination of organic, nonorganic, and biotech farming.

should be constructive. There are profound differences between the principles driving today's GE applications in agriculture versus the principles underlying organic farming. The sooner the public understands these differences and decides which set of principles should shape their food future, the sooner the country can progress toward more coherent national food, farm, and technology policies. Today's muddling serves no one well.

A positive food safety message

There is new information on both the exposure and toxicity side of the pesticide risk assessment equation.

Much new data on pesticide residues in food has emerged as a result of the passage of the Food Quality Protection Act (FQPA) in 1996. This historic bill directed the U.S. EPA [Environmental Protection Agency] to conduct a reassessment of all food uses of pesticides, taking into account the heightened susceptibility of infants and children, the elderly, and other vulnerable population groups.

Why the focus on risks to infants and children? Because kids, especially infants, consume more food per kilogram of bodyweight than adults do and a much less varied diet. As a result, exposure to a pesticide from consumption of a given food is greater per kilogram of infant/child bodyweight compared to adults. Plus, exposure to some pesticides during infancy, even at very low levels, can lead to serious life-long consequences if the pesticides disrupt hormone-driven developmental processes.

In the early 1990s surprisingly little was known about the frequency or levels of pesticides in food as actually eaten. Then-existing government data on residues had been collected as part of tolerance enforcement programs and represented residues at the farm gate, prior to washing, shipping, storage, marketing, and preparation. Relatively insensitive analytical methods were used.

To improve the accuracy of FQPA-driven pesticide dietary risk assessments, Congress funded a new USDA [U.S. Department of Agriculture] program in 1991, the "Pesticide Data Program" (PDP). By design, the PDP focuses on the foods consumed most heavily by children and food is tested, to the extent possible, "as eaten." (A banana or orange samples are tested without the peel; processed foods are tested as they come out of a can, jar or freezer bag.)

Ten years of PDP testing has greatly enhanced understanding of pesticide residues in the United States food supply. About a dozen foods are tested annually. Some 600 to 650 samples are tested of each fresh or processed food, reflecting domestic production and imports roughly proportional to their respective share of overall consumption. Plus, market claims associated with a given food item, such as "organic," "IPM-grown," "No Detectable Residues" or "pesticide free," are recorded roughly in proportion to their occurrence in retail market channels. As a result, PDP results make possible comparison of the distribution and frequency of pesticide residues in domestic versus imported foods, across food groups, as well as comparisons by market claim.

The first-ever analysis of pesticides in organic versus conventional foods was published in the peer-reviewed journal *Food Additives and Contaminants* in early 2002. The paper analyzed six years of PDP data, 10 years of California Department of Pesticide Regulation (DPR) data, and results of Consumers Union testing of four crops. . . .

Pesticide residues in conventional and organic foods

Some major food groups—most oils, dairy, meat, and poultry products—contain few detectable pesticides and contribute very modestly at the national level to dietary exposure and risk. About a dozen pesticides are present routinely in fresh produce and juices derived from produce at levels that pose significant risks, to the extent contemporary risk assessment science and toxicological data accurately reflects real-world risks.

Despite much new data and more refined risk assessment methods, several key children's foods still contain worrisome pesticide residues six years after passage of the FQPA. The foods most likely to contain residues of high-risk pesticides are apples, pears, peaches, grapes, green beans, tomatoes, peas, strawberries, spinach, peppers, melons, lettuce, and various juices.

Nearly three-quarters of the fresh fruits and vegetables (F&V) consumed most frequently by children in the U.S. contain residues and almost half the F&V samples tested from 1994 to 1999 in the PDP contain two or more residues. In general, soft-skinned fruit and vegetables tend to contain residues more frequently than foods with thicker skins, shells, or peels.

The pattern of residues found in organic foods tested by the

PDP differs markedly from the pattern in conventional samples. Conventional fruits are 3.6 times more likely to contain residues than organic fruit samples and conventional vegetables are 6.8 times more likely to have one or more detectable residues.

Compared to organic produce, conventional samples also tend to contain multiple residues much more often. Imported foods consistently contain more residues than domestic samples, regardless of market claim.

Averaged across the PDP and DPR data sets, just under 7 percent of positive organic samples and 54 percent of positive conventional samples contained multiple residues. The average positive conventional apple sample contained 3.2 pesticides, peaches contained 3.1 residues, and celery and cucumber contained 2.7.

Data from DPR testing in 1999 and 2000 shows that conventional food is more than five times more likely to contain residues than organic samples. It is worth noting that organic farmers, processors, and retailers are doing a better job in preventing fraud and pesticide drift [from spraying in nearby fields] and other inadvertent residues, given the downward trend in the frequency of residues in organic foods. In 1996–1998 testing by DPR, just over 12 percent of organic samples tested positive on average, while 7.1 percent contained detectable residues in 1999–2000. There was little change in the frequency of residues in conventional foods, which averaged 38.3 percent annually from 1996–1998 and 40 percent in 1999–2000. . . .

Pesticide toxicity

Implementation of the FQPA triggered an explosion in toxicological and risk assessment research on the developmental effects of pesticides. During fetal development and the first years of life, infants are much less able to detoxify most pesticides and are uniquely vulnerable to developmental toxins, especially neurotoxins, given that the brain and nervous system continue developing through about age 12.

New toxicological data have forced downward by one to two orders of magnitude the allowable levels of exposure to various pesticides found in food. The EPA has had to phase out hundreds of food uses of relatively high-risk pesticides (mostly organophosphate insecticide uses) in order to meet the FQPA's new "reasonable certainty of no harm" standard.

In the last decade much new evidence has emerged on the mechanisms through which pesticides can disrupt development as a result of even very low exposures. . . .

University of California-Berkeley School of Public Health scientists found that exposures to pesticides during pregnancy significantly heightened risk of children developing leukemia and that the more frequent the exposures and the earlier in life, the greater the increase in risk. A team in the Department of Preventive Medicine, University of Southern California, found that exposure to pesticides in the home during fetal development increased the risk of Non-Hodgkin's lymphoma, with odds ratios as high as 9.6 for Burkitt lymphoma.

> *// Scientists found that exposures to pesticides during pregnancy significantly heightened risk of children developing leukemia. //*

A study in Ontario, Canada, confirmed that exposures to pesticides three months prior to conception and during pregnancy increased the risk of spontaneous abortions.

Research supported by the French Ministry of Environment documented clear linkages between exposures to pesticides commonly used in grape vineyards and long-term adverse cognitive effects. Cognitive performance was compared in a group of children living in an upland agricultural region in Mexico where substantial pesticide use occurred, compared to a similar cohort in a nearby village. Children exposed to pesticides had lessened stamina and attention spans, impaired memory and hand-eye coordination, and greater difficulty making simple line drawings.

Just-published work on the developmental neurotoxicity of the most widely used insecticide in the United States, chlorpyrifos, showed that this organophosate (OP) targets [the brain and liver]. The authors conclude that exposures to this OP during the first few years of life are likely a greater risk than during fetal development, although prenatal exposures appear to disrupt the architectural organization of specific regions in the brain and the development of the fetal liver. . . .

The most compelling new study to appear on pesticide dietary risks in a long time was published online on October 31,

2002, in the highly respected journal *Environmental Health Perspectives*. A team based at the University of Washington's School of Public Health and Community Medicine carried out the research. The research assesses the difference in organophosphate (OP) residues and risk faced by two to five year olds consuming a diet composed of mostly organic foods versus conventional foods. . . .

The team found that two to five year olds consuming mostly organic foods over a three day period had much lower mean levels of organophosphate (OP) insecticide metabolites in their urine—in fact, children consuming conventional food had 8.5 times higher average levels than children eating mostly an organic diet. The study was carefully designed to avoid other potential confounding variables. The children came from similar socio-economic backgrounds; households with recent use of pesticides in the home were excluded from the study; and rigorous sampling and double-blind testing protocols were used. The research team also correlated differences in OP metabolite levels to likely risk levels, as measured by the EPA. They concluded that:

> . . . Data suggest that . . . consumption of organic produce represents a relatively simple means for parents to reduce their children's exposure to pesticides.

The pesticide residue data reviewed earlier provides a solid basis to predict a substantial difference in exposure among people consuming largely conventional versus largely organic food. Moreover, it is clear that fresh fruits and vegetables, and fruit juices, account for the lion's share of dietary exposure. [One] study provides the first direct empirical confirmation of this prediction and moreover, supports the encouraging conclusion that by switching to predominantly organic produce and fruit juices, a child's pesticide exposures can be reduced to negligible levels, unlikely to pose significant risks, during this critical period of development.

Organic farmers and consumers are not the only ones that should rejoice at these findings. Conventional farmers adopting biointensive Integrated Pest Management systems can also markedly reduce OP insecticide use. Extensive evidence compiled by the EPA over the course of implementing the FQPA suggests that by cutting out all OP sprays within 90 to 120 days of harvest on major kids' foods, OP residues will largely, if not fully disappear from fresh produce. This is also good news for EPA, which can now confidently predict major progress in reducing OP risks following a relatively small number of regulatory actions targeting less than two-dozen foods.

Why organic food sometimes contains residues

Many people wonder why between 10 percent and one-quarter of organic F&V samples contain residues of synthetic pesticides. Like transgenic DNA, pesticides are ubiquitous and mobile across agricultural landscapes. Most positive organic samples contain low levels of pesticides used on nearby conventional fields. They move onto organic food via drift or through use of contaminated irrigation water. Soil-bound residues of persistent pesticides account for a large portion of residues in root crops and squashes. Cross-contamination with post-harvest fungicides applied in storage facilities is a major cause of low-level fungicide residues. The small percent of samples sold as organic and found to contain relatively high levels of residues likely arise from inadvertent mixing of produce, laboratory error, mislabeling, or fraud.

> *Data suggest that . . . consumption of organic produce represents a relatively simple means for parents to reduce their children's exposure to pesticides.*

A few pro-pesticide activists have gone to great lengths to convince consumers that pesticide residues in organic food are as risky as those in conventional foods. Fortunately, these claims do not pass the laugh test. Expanded residue testing of botanicals and biopesticides would be needed to decisively settle the empirical issues behind such specious claims. Settling this artificial controversy would mean less testing to better understand significant pesticide dietary risks, a tradeoff thus far rejected by government regulatory and research agencies.

It is also true that organic farmers apply non-synthetic pesticides including sulfur, oils, several botanicals, *Bacillus thuringiensis* (*Bt*), soaps, certain microbial pesticides, and pheromones.

By volume, major pesticides used on both organic and conventional farms include sulfur, horticultural/petroleum distillates and oils, and copper-based fungicides. There are some formulations of these pesticides approved for organic production and many others available to conventional growers. These pesticides are used in similar ways for comparable reasons on organic and conventional fruit and vegetable farms. Sulfur is almost certainly the most common pesticide residue present on conventional and organic F&Vs, but it is never tested for because it is exempt from the requirement for a tolerance and poses essentially no risk through the diet. Copper is also not tested for because of tolerance exemptions and the fact that copper is an essential nutrient and harmless at the levels ingested as food residues.

Organic farmers also rely on *Bacillus thuringiensis* insecticides, pheromones, and products that coat produce with nontoxic, biodegradable materials (e.g., soaps and clays). Residues of these pesticides are rarely tested for because there are no tolerances to enforce and no basis for food safety concerns, given how these products are used in production agriculture.

While there were once several toxic botanical insecticides on the market and approved for organic production, only one remains in relatively common use—pyrethrins. Pesticides containing pyrethrins are indeed toxic but they degrade rapidly after spraying and hence rarely leave detectable residues. Plus, they are applied at very low rates, on the order of one to two one-hundredths of a pound per acre; OP insecticides are applied at 50- to 100-times higher rates. Other botanicals of possible concern include rotenone and sabadilla. The most recent survey of organic farmers carried out by the Organic Farming Research Foundation (OFRF) found that only 9 percent of 1,045 farmers applied botanicals regularly (mostly pyrethrins and neem), and that 52 perent never use them, 21 percent use them rarely, and 18 percent "on occasion."

Organic food reduces exposure to pesticides

To the extent consumers become aware of recently published data and research findings on pesticides in food, new information will reinforce already deep-set concerns. It is now clear that purchasing organic food is a reliable way to markedly reduce exposure to pesticides. Less exposure means greater margins of safety. While toxicologists and risk assessment experts will argue until the cows come home over whether 0.05 ppm [parts per million] of pesticide X, Y, or Z is safe or unsafe, many consumers are now looking for practical ways to reduce personal risk loads. Consuming organic food is clearly one way to do just that.

Several times in recent years, the USDA has stated publicly that organic food is no safer than any other food. Even more frequently and assertively, the USDA has claimed that GE foods are fully tested and pose no risks. Bush administration and USDA leaders are puzzled why so many people around the world are not willing to accept the official position of the U.S. government regarding the safety of GE foods. The credibility of the U.S. government, and confidence around the world in food exports from the U.S., rests upon whether food safety conclusions reached by the USDA, and pushed by the government, are grounded in sound science and consistent with the latest research findings. Clearly, the USDA needs to look anew at recent data on pesticide residues in conventional and organic foods and reconsider its message, in the interest of restoring confidence in the Department's scientific abilities and openness to new information.

12

Pesticides Are Rarely Dangerous and Provide Many Benefits

Scott Phillips, Robert Krieger, Michael Goodman, James Lamb, and William Robertson

Scott Phillips serves as associate clinical professor of medicine in the division of clinical pharmacology and toxicology at the University of Colorado Health Sciences Center and is the attending physician at the Rocky Mountain Poison and Drug Center. Robert Krieger is a researcher at the University of California who specializes in chemical risk assessment. Michael Goodman is a pediatrician who specializes in epidemiology. James Lamb is a toxicologist and environmental consultant. William Robertson is a professor of pediatrics at the University of Washington and director of the Seattle Poison Control Center.

Pesticides are sprayed on foods grown in home gardens and on foods served in school cafeterias. While pesticide use poses some risks, there is no statistically significant correlation between low exposure to pesticides and cancer or neurological damage. Doctors, scientists, and pesticide experts agree that the benefits of these chemicals outweigh the harmful effects.

Editor's note: The following selection is the transcript from a panel discussion about pesticide safety, moderated by Scott Phillips.

S cott Phillips: *Among the obvious concerns the public has about pesticides is the potential for poisonings. How serious a problem is pesticide poisoning in terms of both its prevalence and how seriously people and children are hurt?*

Robert Krieger, Ph.D.: I understand the public's concern, but the fact is poisoning from pesticides is a very rare event because of the way they are used. Data from the American Association of Poison Control Centers show that in 2000, 920 deaths were caused by poisonings, including by drugs, medicines, carbon monoxide, mushrooms, snakes, wasps and bees, shellfish and other commonly recognized agents. Compare that to the 20 people who died from pesticide poisonings in 2000, 17 of whom were intentional ingestions. Two of the unintentional deaths were in children who ingested pesticides not typically used in and around schools or buildings; the other, an adult who died from an unknown pesticide. Obviously, we don't want any of these deaths. But the numbers clearly indicate the health threat of pesticide poisoning is usually substantially overestimated. There is a very low likelihood people can be overexposed to these products by normal use.

> *When pesticide use results in harmful effects, the cause is almost inevitably human failure to heed instructions for use.*

Michael Goodman, M.D.: I agree with Dr. Krieger. I'd just like to add that the data indicate parents often contact the poison control centers expressing concerns regarding children's exposures to pesticides. However, 90 percent of these exposures do not require any medical intervention, the numbers of serious poisonings are very small and they are the result of serious and often intentional misuse.

Phillips: *Are these poisonings, however rare, enough of a problem to curtail pesticide use in the schools or elsewhere?*

Krieger: I don't know of any poisoning or health issues resulting from normal use of pesticides in schools. Pesticides are probably used more frequently in children's homes than in schools. Children's exposures represent trace amounts relative to toxic levels. Pesticide use in schools doesn't represent a threat to health.

Goodman: While prevention of poisonings in general is very important, banning pesticides from schools may lead to serious public health consequences such as increased risk of insect-borne and rodent-borne diseases.

Phillips: *Are there important things that schools should do to reduce the likelihood or a problem?*

Goodman: Certainly, and they are quite simple. Potentially effective measures may include avoiding storage of pesticides on school property and scheduling pesticide application when students and staff are not present.

Krieger: Schools should develop and implement a well-conceived integrated pest management plan that makes clear the conditions for pesticide use. This will permit schools to respond promptly when pest problems occur and will provide assurance that there is no needless exposure.

Pesticide safety

Phillips: *We've addressed the issue of poisoning but beyond that, are pesticides a health threat to children? Should parents and public officials be worried about health problems resulting from even minute levels of pesticide exposure?*

James Lamb, Ph.D.: As a toxicologist, I can tell you that properly used pesticides pose no more than minimal everyday risks to adults and children. As with any product, improper use of pesticides can be dangerous. They need to be handled with appropriate respect and care to ensure that they are used safely.

Goodman: High levels of pesticide exposure are unacceptable and potentially dangerous. However, there is no indication from studying years of scientific and medical evidence that appropriate safe use and handling of pesticides pose a health threat to children.

Krieger: Let me just add that over-the-counter pesticides, available to homeowners, are formulated to meet consumer needs in homes and schools. When pesticide use results in harmful effects, the cause is almost inevitably human failure to heed instructions for use.

"Organic" pesticides and pesticide bans

Phillips: *With many so-called "non-toxic" or "organic" pest control options being promoted to consumers, some people may ask why we shouldn't just stop using chemical pesticides altogether?*

Goodman: It is true that many pest control options are being marketed as non-toxic. However, so-called natural pesticides are not necessarily safer than synthetic ones. Animal studies indicate that about one-half of all naturally occurring compounds may be carcinogenic at high doses. Unless and until a natural product is actually tested for carcinogenicity, one cannot predict the results based simply on the fact that it is "natural." Furthermore, organic pesticides may be more expensive and less effective than synthetic pesticides. There is no evidence that banning pesticides will improve public health and help prevent diseases. Most toxins ingested by people are natural. For example, more than 99 percent of the pesticides in our diet are compounds that are naturally present in plants. Some of those naturally occurring chemicals have been shown to cause diseases in laboratory animals at high doses. Nevertheless, humans are exposed to them at low levels on a regular basis and without any adverse health effects.

Lamb: I agree with Dr. Goodman. "Organic" and "natural" are not synonyms for "better" or "safer." All chemicals, including natural chemicals, have the potential to cause harm if they are not properly handled. In some cases, natural products are more dangerous or less effective than their synthetic counterparts. Synthetic products have been designed to improve on nature and to increase effectiveness or decrease the required dose or side effects by using the same chemical mechanisms as natural chemicals to control pests. . . .

Phillips: *But some people are calling for complete bans of pesticides. . . . Why not be "better safe than sorry"?*

William Robertson, M.D.: Let me be frank. Proponents of the so-called "precautionary principle"—the notion that we should ban products and chemicals even in the absence of evidence that they cause harm—have worked very hard to oversell risk. Unfortunately if you believe this theory, you'd never get out of bed in the morning or drive your car. Remember there simply is no certainty of absence or lack of risk in life. Risk can be high or low—but never totally absent. There are significant risks in NOT using pesticides that must be considered. If we are to make sound decisions about pesticides, we simply must get everyone to put aside their "chemophobia" and replace it with a more reasonable, realistic mindset.

Pesticides and health effects

Phillips: *Could a child develop cancer because of exposure to pesticides?*

Krieger: Based on a number of studies during the past 50 years, pesticides aren't any more likely than other classes of chemicals to be potential human carcinogens. It's also highly unlikely since exposures are intermittent and far below toxic thresholds. A child is more likely to get cancer from the sunshine than from the use of pesticides. . . . In everyday life, the most significant environmental cancer risk for children is normal exposure to sunshine.

> *There are significant risks in NOT using pesticides that must be considered.*

Lamb: It is extremely unlikely that normal use of a pesticide could cause cancer in children or adults. A substantial amount of safety data is developed and thoroughly evaluated before the product is approved for use. Product safety study findings are used to set the conditions for use, and the exposures to children are carefully considered in developing the label instructions for pesticide use. Exposures are limited to minimize risk of any adverse health effect to children, including cancer.

Robertson: Allow me to add that current scientific thinking never lets us say never. Instead, science lets us focus on the "likelihood of an event"—a 10-percent risk or a 1-percent risk or an infinitesimal risk—at which point the individual or the society makes a choice. At the present time, as it has been for the past 30 years, science agrees that the risk of pesticides causing any cancer in adults or in children is extremely remote, though such a "risk" can never be said not to exist.

Phillips: *As scientists, we understand the use of laboratory animals to determine product safety. But what should the public think when it hears about scientific studies showing that pesticides cause cancer in laboratory animals?*

Lamb: There is no reason for the public to be concerned. The animal safety studies use high doses for nearly the entire life of the test animal. The very purpose of the studies is to create an adverse effect—to determine how much exposure is necessary to make the animal sick. So, the exposure levels to these chemicals are immense. In some studies, the effect may be cancer. Under these test conditions, even some natural chemicals found in food can cause cancer and other adverse effects. However, we should be less concerned about which effects are observed than about the doses or exposure concentrations that cause the effects and compare them to the levels to which we might be exposed. For pesticides, we find that the dose levels that caused cancer in animals far exceed our exposure levels.

Krieger: We must use great caution when applying the results of animal studies to people's everyday experiences. Let me stress that the high lifetime dosages used in these studies are so extreme that they are difficult to relate to normal living conditions. Pesticides are very unlikely to contribute to cancer due to the nature and limited extent of human pesticide exposures.

Phillips: *During the past few years, the public has read about a new theory called endocrine modulation, or endocrine disruption. A 1999 National Academy of Sciences report on the endocrine disruption hypothesis found little evidence to support allegations about chemicals and adverse effects in people. Do you think that the use of pesticides can harm a child's hormonal system?*

> *Relative rankings do not show pesticide exposure to be particularly high in comparison to everyday risks such as smoking, riding in a car . . . or crossing the street.*

Robertson: After four years of scientific review and debate, the National Research Council Committee on Hormonally Active Agents in the Environment reported that no conclusions could be drawn about potential health effects of low-dose exposures to certain chemicals. Many chemicals have "estrogen-like" effects. In my opinion, endocrine disruption is simply "much ado about nothing." For the most part, humans can tolerate the low level of pesticides found in their environment without any immediate or long-term effects. And, remember, public exposure to naturally occurring, hormonally active substances are at levels millions of times greater than those levels that may be associated with chemical exposures. My bottom line is that it's a provocative theory that the media likes to report on but there's nothing I've seen that suggests people should be concerned about it.

Phillips: *Some advocacy groups have raised new charges, not yet proved through scientific research, that pesticides are a serious threat to brain development and may cause neurological disorders. What's the reaction of the medical community to these reports?*

Goodman: The current scientific literature contains several reports evaluating the relation between environmental chemical exposures and neurobehavioral test scores in children. At the present time, none of these studies has clearly shown an adverse effect of pesticide exposure on the neurodevelopment of children. With the exception of lead poisoning, these studies show little evidence of a consistent adverse effect of chemicals at low levels of exposure. The problems with these types of studies stem from their inability to account for other factors, such as socioeconomic status, childhood disease and nutrition, and maternal substance abuse or poor nutrition during pregnancy. Many of these potential factors are far more powerful predictors of neurodevelopmental problems than the hypothesized environmental exposure to chemicals.

Pesticide testing and regulation

Phillips: *A lot of what we've talked about assumes that pesticides are used properly. What laws and regulations are in place to ensure the proper formulation, distribution and use of pesticides on the farm, in homes and in schools?*

Lamb: The federal government, through the Environmental Protection Agency [EPA] regulates and enforces safe pesticide use. States and local governments cooperate in enforcing federal pesticide laws and regulations and may also have additional requirements. First, before a pesticide can be sold or distributed, it must be tested by the company and approved or registered by EPA. Millions of dollars of toxicology and chemistry data are typically required, under extremely demanding conditions. The primary tool for controlling pesticide use and exposure is the pesticide label. Once the product is registered for a specific use, the user must be certain that the product is approved for the target pest and that the label directions are followed. Some pesticide products are restricted to use by certified applicators as spelled out in the EPA requirements.

Krieger: To add to that, I believe chemicals that are used as pesticides are probably the most thoroughly tested chemicals with respect to their potential to have adverse effects on health or environmental quality. Basic short-term toxicity testing is performed to help establish conditions of use. Longer-term studies determine a chemical's potential to produce effects such as teratogenicity, immunotoxicity, carcinogenicity, mutagenicity and behavioral effects. Possible ecological effects are also part of pesticide testing programs. Taken together, a substantial scientific database is available for regulatory evaluation of pesticide uses.

Phillips: *Given everything we've discussed, how do pesticides rank in terms of threats to public health?*

Lamb: Relative rankings do not show pesticide exposure to be particularly high in comparison to everyday risks such as smoking, riding in a car, exposure to communicable disease or crossing the street. In fact, the ranking of pesticide risk when compared to these other everyday risks is very low.

Robertson: In the opinions of experts and individuals trained in the world of science, the ranking is extraordinarily low. Among the general public, unfortunately, pesticides rank far higher on the risk scale than they should.

Organizations to Contact

The editors have compiled the following list of organizations concerned with the issues debated in this book. The descriptions are derived from materials provided by the organizations. All have publications or information available for interested readers. The list was compiled on the date of publication of the present volume; the information provided here may change. Be aware that many organizations take several weeks or longer to respond to inquiries, so allow as much time as possible.

AgBioWorld Foundation
PO Box 85, Tuskegee, AL 36087-0085
(334) 444-7884
e-mail: prakash@tuskegee.edu • Web site: www.agbioworld.org

The AgBioWorld Foundation is a nonprofit organization that sponsors research into biotechnology, transgenic food, and genetically engineered organisms.

American Council on Science and Health (ACSH)
1995 Broadway, Second Floor, New York, NY 10023-5860
(212) 362-7044 • fax: (212) 362-4919
e-mail: acsh@acsh.org • Web site: www.acsh.org

ACSH provides consumers with scientific evaluations of food and the environment, pointing out both health hazards and benefits. It publishes the bimonthly *News and Views*, as well as the booklets *Eating Safely: Avoiding Foodborne Illness, Biotechnology and Food*, and *Modernize the Food Safety Laws: Delete the Delaney Clause.*

Center for Consumer Freedom
1775 Pennsylvania Ave. NW, Suite 1200, Washington, DC 20006
(202) 463-7110 • fax: (202) 463-7107
e-mail: rberman@new-reality.com
Web site: www.consumerfreedom.com

The Center for Consumer Freedom is a nonprofit coalition supported by restaurants, food companies, and consumers working to promote personal responsibility and protect consumer choices. The center opposes health care advocates, food activists, and politicians who, it believes, are taking away Americans' freedom to eat and drink what they want.

Center for Global Food Issues (CGFI)
PO Box 202, Churchville, VA 24421-0202
(540) 337-6354 • fax: (540) 337-8593
e-mail: www.cgfi.com • Web site: www.cgfi.org/index.htm

The Center for Global Food Issues researches and publishes articles about agriculture and the environmental concerns related to food and fiber production. The center supports genetic engineering, pesticide use, irradiation of food, and other ways of technology in agriculture.

Center for Science in the Public Interest (CSPI)
1875 Connecticut Ave. NW, Suite 300, Washington, DC 20009
(202) 332-9110 • fax: (202) 265-4954
e-mail: cspi@cspinet.org • Web site: www.cspinet.org

The Center for Science in the Public Interest is a consumer advocacy organization whose twin missions are to conduct innovative research and advocacy programs in health and nutrition and to provide consumers with current, useful information about their health and well-being. CSPI supplies information to the public and policy makers and conducts research on food, alcohol, health, the environment, and other issues related to science and technology.

Environmental Working Group (EWG)
1436 U St. NW, Suite 100, Washington, DC 20009
(202) 667-6982
Web site: www.ewg.org

The Environmental Working Group is a nonprofit organization of scientists, engineers, policy experts, lawyers, and computer programmers who research threats to the environment and people's health and look for solutions to environmental problems. In addition, the group lobbies for stronger regulations on the environment.

Food First
398 Sixtieth St., Oakland, CA 94618
(510) 654-4400 • fax: (510) 654-4551
e-mail: foodfirst@foodfirst.org • Web site: www.foodfirst.org

Food First is a member-supported, nonprofit progressive think tank and education center. Its goal is to find solutions to hunger and poverty around the world. Food First publishes books, reports, articles, and films, and provides a variety of lectures, workshops, and academic courses for the public and policy makers.

Food Safety and Inspection Service (FSIS)
1400 Independence Ave. SW, Room 2932-S, Washington, DC 20250-3700
(202) 720-7943 • fax: (202) 720-1843
e-mail: fsiswebmaster@usda.gov • Web site: www.fsis.usda.gov

The Food Safety and Inspection Service is the public health agency of the U.S. Department of Agriculture responsible for ensuring that the nation's commercial supply of meat, poultry, and egg products is safe, wholesome, and correctly labeled and packaged. It publishes fact sheets, reports, articles, and brochures on food safety topics.

Food Safety Consortium (FSC)
110 Agriculture Building, University of Arkansas
Fayetteville, AR 72701
(501) 575-5647 • fax: (501) 575-7531
e-mail: fsc@cavern.uark.edu • Web site: www.uark.edu/depts/fsc

Congress established the Food Safety Consortium, consisting of researchers from the University of Arkansas, Iowa State University, and

Kansas State University, in 1988 through a special Cooperative State Research Service grant. It conducts extensive investigation into all areas of poultry, beef, and pork meat production. The consortium publishes the quarterly *FSC Newsletter*.

Friends of the Earth (FOE)
1717 Massachusetts Ave. NW, Suite 600, Washington, DC 20036-2002
(877) 843-8687 • fax: (202) 783-0444
e-mail: foe@foe.org • Web site: www.foe.org

Friends of the Earth monitors legislation and regulations that affect the environment. Its Safer Food, Safer Farms Campaign speaks out against what it perceives as the negative impact biotechnology can have on farming, food production, genetic resources, and the environment. It publishes the quarterly newsletter *Atmosphere* and the magazine *Friends of the Earth* ten times a year.

Harvard Center for Risk Analysis (HCRA)
718 Huntington Ave., Boston, MA 02115
(617) 432-4497 • fax: (617) 432-0190
e-mail: dropeik@hsph.harvard.edu • Web site: www.hcra.harvard.edu

The Harvard Center for Risk Analysis is an organization of biotechnology companies, large food processors, and chemical, pesticide, and petroleum manufacturers. The center analyzes and evaluates the potential risks posed by agricultural and medical technology.

Hudson Institute
1015 Eighteenth St. NW, Suite 300, Washington, DC 20036
(202) 223-7770 • fax: (202) 223-8537
e-mail: info@hudsondc.org • Web site: www.hudson.org

The Hudson Institute is a conservative think tank that provides research, books, and policy recommendations to leaders in communities, businesses, nonprofit organizations, and governments. The institute is committed to free markets and individual responsibility, confidence in the power of technology to assist progress, respect for the importance of culture and religion in human affairs, and determination to preserve America's national security.

National Cattlemen's Beef Association (NCBA)
5420 S. Quebec St., Greenwood Village, CO 80111-1905
(303) 694-0305 • fax: (303) 694-2851
e-mail: cattle@beef.org • Web site: www.beef.org

National Cattlemen's Beef Association is the marketing organization and trade association for America's 1 million cattle farmers and ranchers. Its publications include *The Cattle and Beef Handbook*, *National Cattlemen Magazine*, and *The Beef Business Bulletin*.

Organic Consumers Association (OCA)
6101 Cliff Estate Rd., Little Marais, MN 55614
(218) 226-4164 • fax: (218) 353-7652
Web site: www.organicconsumers.org

The Organic Consumers Association is a nonprofit public interest organization that deals with issues of food safety, industrial agriculture, genetic engineering, corporate accountability, and environmental sustainability. The OCA is the only organization in the United States focused exclusively on representing the views and interests of the nation's estimated 10 million organic consumers.

Public Citizen
215 Pennsylvania Ave. SE, Washington, DC 20003
(202) 546-4996 • fax: (202) 547-7392
e-mail: cmep@citizen.org • Web site: www.citizen.org/cmep

Public Citizen is a national, nonprofit consumer advocacy organization founded in 1971 to represent consumer interests. Public Citizen fights for democratic accountability in government, the right of consumers to seek redress in the courts, safe and sustainable energy sources, fair trade policies, strong environmental protections, and affordable prescription drugs and health care.

U.S. Food and Drug Administration (FDA)
5600 Fishers Ln., Rockville, MD 20857
(888) 463-6332
e-mail: webmail@oc.fda.gov • Web site: www.fda.gov

The FDA is a public health agency, charged with protecting American consumers by enforcing the federal Food, Drug, and Cosmetic Act and several related public health laws. To carry out this mandate of consumer protection, FDA has investigators and inspectors cover the country's almost ninety-five thousand FDA-regulated businesses. Its publications include government documents, reports, fact sheets, and press announcements.

Bibliography

Books

Peter Cox
You Don't Need Meat. New York: Thomas Dunne, 2002.

Greg Critser
Fat Land: How Americans Became the Fattest People in the World. Boston: Houghton Mifflin, 2003.

Gail A. Eisnitz
Slaughterhouse: The Shocking Story of Greed, Neglect, and Inhumane Treatment Inside the U.S. Meat Industry. Amherst, NY: Prometheus, 1997.

Francis Fukuyama
Our Posthuman Future: Consequences of the Biotechnology Revolution. New York: Farrar, Straus and Giroux, 2002.

Michael Fumento
The Fat of the Land: The Obesity Epidemic and How Overweight Americans Can Help Themselves. New York: Viking, 1997.

Myrna Chandler Goldstein
Controversies on Food and Nutrition. Westport, CT: Greenwood, 2002.

Mary Heersink
E. Coli 0157: The True Story of a Mother's Battle with a Killer Microbe. Far Hills, NJ: New Horizon, 1996.

Kathiann M. Kowalski
The Debate over Genetically Engineered Food: Healthy or Harmful? Berkeley Heights, NJ: Enslow, 2002.

Howard Lyman
Mad Cowboy: Plain Truth from the Cattle Rancher Who Won't Eat Meat. New York: Scribner, 1998.

Marion Nestle
Safe Food: Bacteria, Biotechnology, and Bioterrorism. Berkeley: University of California Press, 2003.

Thomas Hugh Pennington
When Food Kills: BSE, E. Coli, and Disaster Science. New York: Oxford University Press, 2003.

Susanna Hornig Priest
A Grain of Truth: The Media, the Public, and Biotechnology. Lanham, MD: Rowman & Littlefield, 2001.

Peter Pringle
Food, Inc.: Mendel to Monsanto—the Promises and Perils of the Biotech Harvest. New York: Simon & Schuster, 2003.

Sheldon Rampton
Mad Cow USA: Could the Nightmare Happen Here? Monroe, ME: Common Courage, 1997.

Jeremy Rifkin
Beyond Beef: The Rise and Fall of the Cattle Culture. New York: Dutton, 1992.

George Ritzer — *The McDonaldization of Society.* Thousand Oaks, CA: Pine Forge, 2000.

Cynthia A. Roberts — *The Food Safety Information Handbook.* Westport, CT: Oryx, 2001.

Eric Schlosser — *Fast Food Nation: The Dark Side of the All-American Meal.* New York: Perennial, 2002.

Jeffrey M. Smith — *Seeds of Deception: Exposing Industry and Government Lies About the Safety of the Genetically Engineered Foods You're Eating.* Fairfield, IA: Yes, 2003.

Mark Jerome Walters — *Six Modern Plagues and How We Are Causing Them.* Washington, DC: Island Press, 2003.

Periodicals

Hannah Beech, Meenakshi Ganguly, and Nelly Sindayen — "Grains of Hope," *Time International*, February 12, 2001.

Marian Burros — "Is Organic Food Provably Better?" *New York Times*, July 16, 2003.

Sean Cavanagh — "Public Awareness Urged on Irradiated Beef in Schools," *Education Week*, January 14, 2004.

Melissa Daly — "Going 'Crunchy': Years Ago, Organic Food Was for Hippies. Today, It's Totally Mainstream. But Is It Really Better for You?" *Seventeen*, March 2003.

Friends of the Earth — "Into the Mouths of Babes: Pesticides in the Diet and Our Children's Health," *Real Food*, March 2002.

George Gray, Joshua Cohen, and Silvia Kreindel — "Evaluating the Risk of Bovine Spongiform Encephalopathy in the United States," *Risk in Perspective*, March 2002.

Stephen Handelman — "An Edible Threat: A Porous Border Means Taking Agricultural Terrorism Seriously," *Time International*, July 28, 2003.

Michael Janofsky — "Where the Slaughterhouse Ruled, a Recall and a Shift in the Wind," *New York Times*, July 22, 2002.

Barbara Keeler — "A Nation of Lab Rats," *Sierra*, July 2001.

John Kepner — "Studies Show Benefits of Eating Organic," *Pesticides and You*, vol. 23, no. 1, 2003.

Brad Knickerbocker — "Risk of Terrorism to Nation's Food Supply: New Research Shows How Easily Livestock and Crops Could Be Hit by 'Agroterrorists,'" *Christian Science Monitor*, December 24, 2002.

Ben Lilliston — "Farmers Fight to Save Organic Crops," *Progressive*, September 2001.

Mac Margolis	"A Mix-Up in Priorities: By Lavishing Money on Cures for Bioterror Attack, America Ignores Prosaic Diseases That Kill Millions," *Newsweek International*, April 5, 2004.
David Martosko	"Food Fetish," *American Spectator*, February 24, 2003.
Rosie Mestel	"Altered Vegetable States," *Discover*, January 1993.
Judith Miller	"Censored Study on Bioterror Doubts U.S. Preparedness," *New York Times*, March 29, 2004.
Steve Mitchell	"Groups Allege Irradiated Food Unsafe," United Press International, October 8, 2002.
Michael Satchell and Stephen J. Hedges	"The Next Bad Beef Scandal: Cattle Feed Now Contains Things like Chicken Manure and Dead Cats," *U.S. News & World Report*, September 1, 1997.
Cindy Skrzycki	"Approval of Irradiated Sweet Potatoes Has Critics Steamed," *Washington Post*, March 9, 2004.
Shankar Vedantam	"U.S. Recalls Meat Linked to Wash. Slaughterhouse; Mad Cow Fears Lead Growing List of Nations to Halt Beef Imports," *Washington Post*, December 25, 2003.

Internet Sources

Alex A. Avery	"Crying Wolf over Mad Cow," Hudson Institute, February 10, 2004. www.hudson.org/index.cfm?fuseaction=publication_details&id=3227.
Dennis Avery	"Can Organic Produce Reduce Children's Pesticide Levels?" Center for Global Food Issues, www.cgfi.org/materials/articles/2003/apr_14_03.htm.
Peter Chalk	"Hitting America's Soft Underbelly: The Potential Threat of Deliberate Biological Attacks Against the U.S. Agricultural and Food Industry," RAND Corporation, 2004. www.rand.org.
Annette Colby	"Is Organic More Nutritious?" Power Nutrition Healthy Eating, www.power-nutrition.com/healthy%20eating/organic.html.
Consumer Policy Institute	"Consumer Reports Finds Pesticide Residues Too High on Some Domestic and Imported Produce," Consumers Union, February 18, 1999. www.consumersunion.org/food/pestny899.htm.
Caroline Smith DeWaal and Kristina Barlow	"Outbreak Alert! 2002," Center for Science in the Public Interest, September 2002. www.cspinet.org/reports/outbreak_report.pdf.

Lawrence J. Dyckman   "Bioterrorism: A Threat to Agriculture and the Food Supply," U.S. General Accounting Office, November 19, 2003. www.gao.gov/new.items/d04259t.pdf.

Environmental Working Group   "BodyBurden: The Pollution in People," 2003. www.ewg.org/issues/home.php?i=6.

Environmental Working Group   "Why Reducing Pesticide Exposure Is Smart," 2004. www.foodnews.org/reduce.php.

National Research Council   "Pesticides in the Diets of Infants and Children," National Academy Press, 1993. http://books.nap.edu/books/0309048753/html/R1.html.

U.S. Department of Agriculture   "The Animal and Plant Health Inspection Service and Department of Homeland Security: Working Together to Protect Agriculture," Animal and Plant Health Inspection Service, May 2003. www.aphis.usda.gov/lpa/pubs/fsheet_faq_notice/fs_aphis_homeland.html.

Index

agribusiness industry
  food poisoning and, 10–11
  methods used by, 7
agricultural terrorism
  awareness of, after September
    11, 24–26
  cases of, 15, 19–21, 24–25
  economic effects of, 17–19
  efforts to counter, 23
  environmental activists and,
    16–17, 19–20
  federal agencies are protecting
    against, 24–32
  food supply is vulnerable to,
    14–23
  reasons for lack of, 19–21
  reducing threat from, 16
  threatens jobs, 17–19
  types of attacks and, 22–23
Americans
  demand for organic food by,
    72–76
  food consumption of, 7
Animal and Plant Health
  Inspection Services (APHIS), 48
animal wastes, 56–58
anthrax attacks, 14
antibiotic resistance, 46
Avery, Alex, 12
Avery, Dennis, 8

Bacillus thuringiensis (Bt),
  103–104
Barlow, Kristina, 10–11
beef supply
  safety of, 11–13
  see also mad cow disease
Benbrook, Charles M., 46–47, 96
Biosafety Protocol, 50
biotechnology. *See* genetically
  engineered (GE) foods
Bioterrorism Act, 28–29
bovine spongiform
  encephalopathy (BSE). *See* mad
  cow disease
Britain

foot-and-mouth disease in,
    15–17
  mad cow disease in, 56
Bruhn, Christine, 77–78

cancer
  irradiated food causes, 80–81
  pesticides and, 109–11
cannibalism disease, 55
canola, 42–43
Cartagena Protocol, 39
cattle-derived feed, 56–59
Center for Consumer Freedom,
  75
Chalk, Peter, 16–17
Charman, Karen, 41
chemical compounds, in
  irradiated food, 82–84
children, pesticides effect on, 8,
  98–102, 106–11
Chilean grape poisoning, 15
chronic wasting disease (CWD),
  57–58
Codex Alimentarius
  Commission, 85–86
Coleman, Mel, Jr., 76
Coleman Natural Beef, 76–77
Conko, Gregory, 33
corn, 42–43
cotton, 42–43
Creutzfeldt-Jakob disease (CJD),
  12, 55, 64
crop diversity, GE foods and, 50
Cummings, Ronnie, 75

Department of Health and
  Human Services (HHS), 25
developing countries, growth of
  GE foods in, 34–35
DeWaal, Caroline Smith, 10–11
DiMotta, Katherine, 75
Dunn, Michael, 18

E. coli infections, 69–70
economic costs, of agricultural
  terrorism, 17–19

122

Eden Foods, 49–50
Ellstrand, Norman C., 51
environment
  benefits to, of GE foods, 35–37
  effects of GE foods on, 46–48
  irradiated food and, 90, 92
Environmental Protection
  Agency (EPA), 112
environmental terrorism, 19–20
  see also agricultural terrorism

Farm Bill, 94
farmers, effects of GE foods on,
  48–50
Flavr Savr tomatoes, 8–9
food-borne illnesses, irradiation
  and, 87–92
food consumption, of
  Americans, 7
food imports, FDA regulation of,
  27–28, 30
food irradiation. *See* irradiated
  food
food poisoning, 10–11
Food Quality Protection Act
  (FQPA), 98
food supply
  demand for information about,
  72–73
  federal agencies are protecting,
  24–32
  insect infestation of, 89
  irradiation of
    is unsafe, 79–86
    makes it safer, 87–95
  is vulnerable to agricultural
    terrorism, 14–23
  pesticides in
    are poisoning consumers,
    96–105
    are safe, 106–13
  vulnerability of, 21–23
foot-and-mouth disease, 15–17

genetically engineered (GE)
  foods
  approval of, by FDA, 8–9
  are safe and beneficial, 33–40
  changes made to, 43–44
  contamination of native plants
    by, 47–48
  effects of, on farmers, 48–50
  environmental benefits of,
    35–37
  environmental effects of, 46–48
  first appearance of, 8–9
  improve nutritional benefits,
    37–38
  labeling of, 9–10, 50
  vs. organic foods, 36
  patents on, 50
  potential harm from, 41–51
  prevalence of, 43
  restrictions on, 39
  safety concerns about, 9–10,
    44–46
  Terminator technology and,
    43–44
  threaten crop diversity, 50
  unanswered questions about,
    42–43
  will help end hunger, 33–35,
    37–38
genetically modified organisms
  (GMOs)
  genetic structure of, 45–46
  release of, into environment,
    42
Glickman, Dan, 68
Golden Rice, 37, 43
Goodman, Michael, 106
Gray, George, 60
Greco, Jeff, 14

Hansen, Michael, 45
Harvard Center for Risk Analysis
  (HCRA), 58–61
Hatfield, Doc, 72–73, 78
health benefits, of GE foods,
  37–38
health problems
  antibiotic resistance and, 46
  caused by irradiated foods,
    79–86
  caused by pesticides, 96–105
  are overrated, 106–13
herbicides. *See* pesticides
Hoffman, Bruce, 16–17
hunger, GE foods will help end,
  37–38

Idell, William C., 87
India, GE foods in, 34–35
infective prions, 53–56, 65
Integrated Pest Management
  systems, 102

irradiated food
  approval of, 84–85, 93–94
  causes health problems, 79–86
  controversy over, 94–95
  environmental advantages of,
    90
  food-borne illnesses and, 87–92
  international objections to,
    85–86
  is safer, 87–95
  labeling of, 93
  nutritional consequences of,
    90–91
  process of, 88
  toxic chemicals in, 82–84
  worker safety and, 92–93

Jacobsen, Janet, 49

Kanik, Audrey L. Anastasia, 87
Kirschenmann, Fred, 49
Knapp, Alex, 67
Krieger, Robert, 106
kuru, 55

Lacey, Richard, 45
Lamb, James, 106
Lichtenstein, Alice H., 87

MacGuire, Dan, 48–49
mad cow disease, 11–13
  demand for organic food and,
    72–75
  effects of, on beef
    consumption, 77–78
  HCRA study on, 58–61
  rendering and, 56–58
McCammon, Sally, 48
meat and bone meal (MBM),
  56–59
meat industry
  destructive nature of, 52–53
  organic food and, 76–78
  prions, 53–56
  rendering by, 56–58
  see also beef supply; mad cow
    disease
Murphy, Richard McGill, 71

National Cattlemen's Beef
  Association, 59–60, 75
native plants, contamination of,
  47–48

neurological disorders, pesticides
  and, 111–12

obesity, 7
Office of Regulatory Affairs
  (ORA), 27
Operation Liberty Shield, 29–31
Oregon Country Beef, 73
organic farming
  contamination of, 49–50
  vs. GE crops, 36
  pesticides and, 68–69, 96–97,
    108–109
organic food
  beef industry and, 76–78
  consumer demand for, 72–76
  food industry and, 75–76
  is not healthier, 69–70
  is safer and healthier, 71–78
  labeling of, 74
  negative aspects of, 67–70
  pesticide residues in, 99–100,
    103–104
  reduces exposure to pesticides,
    104–105

Parnes, Robin Brett, 87
Pesticide Data Program (PDP),
  98–99
pesticides
  are not dangerous, 106–13
  are poisoning consumers,
    96–105
  bans on, 109
  benefits of, 106–13
  effects of, on children, 8,
    98–102, 106–11
  GE foods require less, 35
  GE foods require more, 46–47
  importance of, 8
  organic, 68–69, 108–109
  organic food reduces exposure
    to, 104–105
  residues of, in foods, 7–8,
    99–100, 103–104
  testing and regulation of,
    112–13
  toxicity of, 100–103
Phillips, Scott, 106
polyploidy, 80
Potter, Michael, 50
Prakash, C.S., 33
Precautionary Principle, 39

Pringle, Peter, 9–10
prions, 53–56, 65
produce, pesticides on, 7–8,
    99–100, 103–104
Prusiner, Stanley, 54–55, 61
Public Citizen, 79
Public Health Security and
    Bioterrorism Preparedness and
    Response Act, 26
Pusztai, Arpad, 46

Race, Rick, 57–58
Rampton, Sheldon, 56
rendering, 56–58
Rifkin, Jeremy, 42
Robertson, William, 106

safety concerns
    about GE foods, 9–10, 44–46
    are unfounded, 33–40
    about irradiated foods, 91–93
slaughterhouses, 11–13
soybeans, 42–43
Stauber, John, 56, 61

Terminator technology, 43–44
terrorism. *See* agricultural
    terrorism
Thompson, Tommy G., 25
transgenic foods. *See* genetically
    engineered (GE) foods
transmissible spongiform
    encephalopathies (TSEs), 54–55,
    57–58
2-ACBs, 83

U.S. Department of Agriculture
    (USDA)

function of, 7
on GE foods, 105
testing of beef by, 60–61, 64
U.S. Food and Drug
    Administration (FDA), 24
approval of GE foods by, 8–9
approval of irradiated food by,
    84–85, 93–94
enforcement of feed ban by,
    58–59
food inspections by, 10–11
food security strategy of, 25–27
function of, 7
is protecting food supply,
    24–32
lack of testing by, on GE foods,
    44–45
Operation Liberty Shield and,
    29–31
regulation of imports and,
    27–28
United States
    mad cow disease in
        is inevitable, 52–62
        is not a threat, 63–66
    obesity in, 7

variant Creutzfeldt-Jakob Disease
    (vCJD), 12, 55, 64
vitamin A deficiency, 37

Walters, Mark Jerome, 11
Wenc, Christine, 52
Whelan, Elizabeth, 63
wildlife habitats, GE foods and,
    36
World Health Organization
    (WHO), 84, 91–92